SURVIVAL HANDBOOK OF MEDICINE AND MEDICAL EMERGENCIES

PREPPER'S OFF-GRID ESSENTIAL GUIDE TO SAVING A LIFE

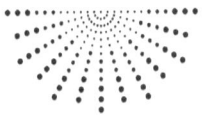

J. B. MAXWELL

CONTENTS

information contained within this document, including, but not limited to, errors, omissions, or inaccuracies.

❀ Created with Vellum

INTRODUCTION

It is not the strongest or the most intelligent who will survive but those who can best manage change. –Leon C. Megginson

---

The feeling that we get while sipping our hot mugs of coffee and lounging on the couch with the warmth of a fire crackling close is that of belonging and security. We rarely consider what life would be like if we didn't have the conveniences of home and medical care. It's strange to think about how quickly things may go wrong and how we could be fighting for our lives alone. Don't you think that's a little scary? Many people have encountered comparable difficulties in the past and have triumphed. The fact is, the world is full of chaos, but the chaos can be managed. The only question is: Are you prepared?

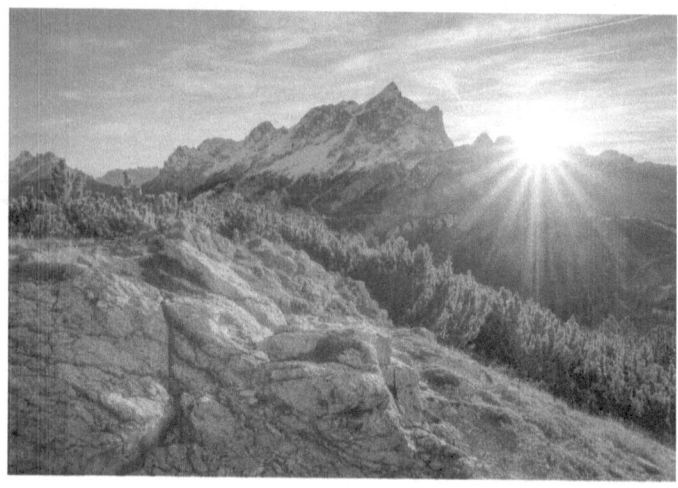

Most of us have heard the story of *Robinson Crusoe* by Daniel Defoe. In simple terms, the whole point of the novel revolved around survival. Similarly, there have been numerous instances in a non-fictional reality where we have heard of people overcoming difficult conditions in the wilderness without access to medical assistance. In one such astonishing incident, Jose Salvador Alvarenga was discovered on the shores of the Marshall Islands' Ebon Atoll in recent years, specifically in 2014. He was said to have been wandering alone in the Pacific

Ocean for 13 months. He had gone on a fishing expedition with a friend with extremely minimal supplies, but he had been blown to an unexpected location due to a severe storm. His boat was also damaged, and his partner died in the tragedy. Jose, on the other hand, managed to survive by eating whatever he could find, including fish, turtles, and birds. He also drank his urine to stay hydrated. The moral that we can take from this story is that if you have the desire to survive in a difficult situation and the necessary expertise to deal with medical issues, you can accomplish anything.

The various pandemics that have struck the globe over time, as well as natural calamities that have wreaked havoc in a variety of ways, have caused us to question our capacity as humans to a large extent. There are moments when we feel powerless and believe that modern medical treatments are the only option to ensure our long-term survival. Even if there is a desire to learn about medicine, there are complexities and problems associated with the educational approach. In emergency situations, it is all the more distressing for someone who wants to study the fundamentals of medicine to deal with medical emergencies before they've had a chance to be medically trained. More so, the sense of powerlessness that comes from seeing someone close to you suffer and not being able to help them, can become a deep-seated source of irritation for the rest of your life.

This book makes a concerted effort to assist anyone who has had a firsthand experience wishing to help a person in agony but was unable to do so due to a lack of medical knowledge. The main goal is to reach as many people as possible to teach them something that will help them survive in difficult circumstances, such as surviving in the wilderness without any professional medical assistance. The methodical approach will provide a precise and in-depth understanding of how a person who has suffered a physical or medical trauma might receive lifesaving first aid help.

No matter how pleasant your current circumstances are, you are still vulnerable to life-changing events. As a result, upgrading your skills and preparing yourself for any type of threat is always a sensible move. Without access to a suitable professional space, you should constantly be informed on how the human body functions and the various therapies that can be administered. It doesn't matter if you're a novice or an expert; the drive to survive is what binds your will and, as a result, your actions.

Learning the techniques and abilities associated with medicinal approaches can provide you with a sense of independence that can be a life-changing experience.

Nature's grandeur cannot be ignored, and the more we study about it, the less we believe we know about it. As a result, we all must work together with nature to nurture, protect, and learn from it. The importance of nature and its various manifestations in the wilderness cannot be overstated. When things go wrong, it may be as unwelcoming as it is challenging. An ultimate survivor is defined by the endurance required to remain safe and sound within their boundaries without the assistance of even the most remote civilization. The skills that you'll learn through this book will not only help you in the outdoors but will equally help you attend to anyone in dire condition.

What if I told you that if you develop your skills and become a medical asset, you can get through even the most terrible situations? Trust me; I've upskilled my knowledge by traveling to different regions of the Far East and discovering jewels of Eastern Medicine including Traditional Chinese and Ayurvedic practices, in addition to the knowledge I've gained over the years from studying within the domains of Western medicine. It is a fact that off-grid living provides a level of comfort and gratitude that is unfathomable. Off-grid living, however, also requires the tools and information needed to medically sustain yourself and those around you.

The primary purpose of this book is to make everyone feel secure and empowered. Because I've spent the last 10 years living in the wilderness and learning survival skills, I believe now is the ideal time to help those who, by choice or by circumstance, find themselves in the wild with no access to medical support. The forests and mountains have a lot to offer, and it's up to us to make the most of it while remaining environmentally conscious. I've witnessed firsthand how nerve-wracking some situations can be, and how, with a little tact, calm can be achieved.

Consider this scenario: You're on vacation and camping out in the woods with your family when you realize you've lost your way back home. The scenario becomes even more difficult for the person who is responsible for the other family members. In such a case, the pressure that builds up can aggravate the condition even more. However, if you have properly prepared yourself for wilderness survival, trust me when I say that you can easily aid your family members and yourself to overcome what could otherwise be a disastrous scenario.

Be it in the wilderness or even in the safe surroundings at your home, anyone could face any form of a medical emergency. Numerous people have preexisting health conditions and allergies which could affect someone's condition all of a sudden. More so, when you are outdoors away from the comforts of home, several causes could lead your health to fall in minutes. What if you are bitten by a snake or a dangerous insect, tumble off a cliff and break your leg, sprain your hands while carrying your heavy pack, suffer frostbite in the chilly mountain regions, or your nose suddenly begins bleeding and won't stop? The point is that medical emergencies can occur at any moment and in any location, and the only way to cope with them is to be prepared!

Many parents are concerned about taking their children on a prolonged vacation due to a lack of medical assistance near the vacation destination. Such anxieties are not uncommon; however, medical emergencies are also fairly uncommon. Therefore, such sentiments should not prevent a person from living the life of their dreams and embarking on a fun-filled adventure wherever. As a result, obtaining a basic understanding of medicine and its purpose, as well as a smattering of wilderness education, is a prerequisite.

Health and safety are the most important concerns for everybody, and via this book, I hope to take you on an enjoyable trip learning about medicine and outdoor survival techniques. I understand that many of us detest reading about medicine because of the complicated medical words. This will not be the case here; you will be able to learn about medicine simply, comprehend the power of natural medicine, understand human anatomy, common injuries, health difficulties, and the different ways to keep trauma at bay in such situations. As a result, with my comprehensive coaching, be prepared to meet a confident and knowledgeable version of yourself. So, let's get started on your journey to becoming a valuable medical asset in any situation.

ARE YOU PREPARED?

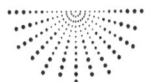

How many of us can say that we dreamed of being a doctor at some point in our life, or to be more specific, during our childhood? So much so that our excitement didn't stop with our confirmation given to the respective teachers at school; it also involved lugging the children's doctor playset around the house and placing a plastic stethoscope around our tiny necks, where we ended up taking everyone's pretend temperature. Furthermore, while many of us have achieved our goals, others have consciously chosen different courses in life that they prefer. The point is that no matter what job we all excel in, knowing a tad bit about medicine and comprehending how to function as a doctor in a medical emergency is something that we all need to know. The primary question remains: How can you be prepared for situations where there is no one to aid you, and you must treat and preserve another person's life as best you can? In other words, let me walk you through how to "be the doctor" in situations where you don't have access to any medical expertise.

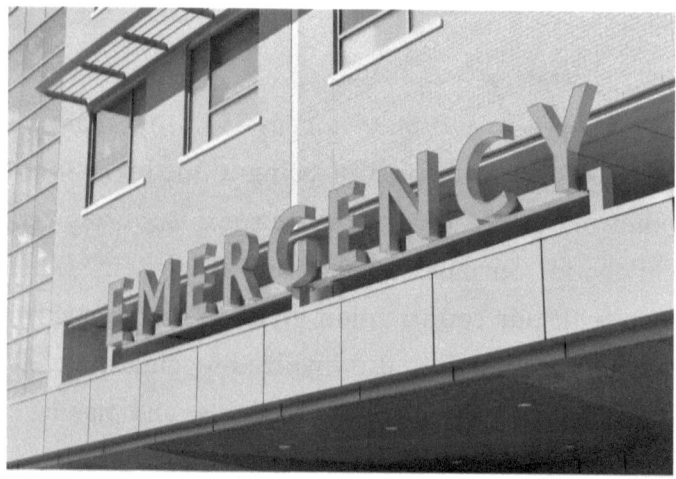

We live in a time when technological and medical developments are at an all-time high. Professionally, people appear to be more preoccupied with work and all of the factors that go along with it. The rush and commotion of city life, as well as our roundtrip commute from work to the office, appear to have taken up the most room in our lives. We are all so preoccupied with catering for the everyday amenities that we forget that there is a world out there in the wilderness that we could visit eventually, either by choice or owing to circumstances. As a consequence, one should consistently be prepared for the best- or worst-case scenario. Not only should you be aware of the situation, but you should also be prepared to learn about medicine, medical emergencies, and, most importantly, how to survive in the wilderness. So, how can you be certain that you will be able to endure adverse circumstances? Well, that takes effort, and in this book, I'll explain to you how to educate yourself and keep abreast of some of the most prominent impediments that people encounter in times of hardship.

We learn the hard way, as they say, and the lessons we learn the hard way may well be the best teaching force for any of us. I've spent over a decade living outdoors, and there have been periods when I've questioned my ability to save those I care about from a potentially dangerous situation. Call it dread or the imprint that certain events left on my mind, nevertheless I decided to learn and study the extensive knowledge of medicine and medical emergencies, as well as to learn the ways of the wild via experience.

Allow me to relay an experience that I have personally witnessed. A group of our friends planned to go on a mountain hiking expedition. We were all looking forward to the experience, despite the difficult ascent. After days of planning and gathering provisions for the long trip and camp fun, we decided to start the adventure. It's hard to convey how exciting the road trip was. We rode across town to the mountain, singing and laughing the whole way. After nearly two days, we arrived at the base of the forest.

The zigzags of the seemingly never-ending trail toward the camp base were tiring, but we were all ecstatic. We were a group of five buddies from various professional backgrounds and had taken several such trips in the past. At the start of the trip, we were given the option of hiring a guide who was familiar with basic paramedic practices and the terrain. However, we refused since we did not want an extra person to make things odd for us while we were having fun. We were five physically robust men who were unafraid of the forest's mysteries. We were so excited that we immediately began our hike.

The first day was fantastic; we opted to camp near a valley that night and began preparing our tent. One of us commenced with the ropes and nails, while the others began preparing meals beside the fire. As we lay in our sleeping bags, gazing up at the sky filled with stars, it was a beautiful night. We fell asleep without even attentively fixing up the tent. We heard one of our friends yell in the early hours of the morning. A shout that could jolt anyone out of their slumber! We rushed toward him to figure out that he was indeed in some excruciating pain. All we could see on his calves was a red rash that looked like a bad bug bite. The place where we had put up for the night was an open space and we had not even imagined that he could have been bitten by a venomous snake in the dark.

Much to my dismay, I didn't consider that it could have been a snake bite at night. We'd heard of and dealt with insect bites before, so we assumed it was such a bite and started using whatever antiseptic cream we had on hand to assist with decreasing the bite's effect. With the daylight setting in, when I looked closely at the red part of his calves, I noticed that it was much more than an insect bite and was possibly a snake bite. It wasn't long after I told my buddies about my doubt that a panic set in. We were befuddled and terrified; we had no clue how to go about treating it, even as a first aid procedure. There was a problem, and our friend, who had been lying down since the dark, was dizzy, sweating, and appeared to be suffering a nervous breakdown. His foot had become fully swelled and inflexible. The agonizing scream that he let out is still fresh in my mind. We attempted everything we could to contact the ranger's post to plead for help. Fortunately, one of our pals was able to make contact with someone at the post and arranged an immediate medical rescue for our friend.

When we arrived at the paramedic station, the doctor noticed that he had become unsteady and that the venom had already caused severe harm to his system. He inquired if we had given him any kind of first aid, and just that question was enough to make my head spin! The point is that when the doctor explained how and what we should have done, even something as easy as taking off his anklet from his foot, something we had never considered, a tinge of guilt lingered in my mind. I believed that if I had some knowledge of recognizing a medical issue and taking the necessary steps to treat it or, at the very least, prevent it from worsening, my friend would not have suffered that miserably.

This encounter shattered my mindset to its core. Things that I had previously dismissed as insignificant were no longer so, which may sound philosophical, but being prepared, knowledgeable, and ready to be a trusted expert, is also a mindset. I was surprised to learn that after a snake bite, any tight objects in a person's clothing should be removed, that if vomit persists, the patient should be kept on their left side to ease them, that their breathing should be closely monitored, and that pressure pads could be used in many cases. I listened to all this information from the doctor and other staff, and only one thing struck my mind: I realized that we had not done a single action of the mentioned first aid steps to help our friend who was yelling even in a subconscious state with pain. This incident made me recognize the value of medical knowledge. I felt it was past due for me to devote more time to researching medical emergencies and wilderness survival. The feeling of helplessness when you see a living being in front of you in agonizing pain and you're unable to help them in any way is the worst that one can feel in their life. My point is, not everyone needs to learn the hard way; you can always be prepared for any difficult situation like this by expanding your knowledge. If we consider similar situations, we may be sure that there are many more people around us who have felt helpless or, more accurately, caught up in a medical emergency. All you can do as an individual is become self-sufficient to the point where you won't be afraid when you're out in the woods or if an emergency arises.

Medicine has been a boon to mankind's well-being as well as the well-being of all living things on the planet. My personal experience and close encounters with problems taught me the importance and depth of comprehending medical information, which fueled my desire to learn more about it. Let me take you through this journey of understanding medicine and its benefits.

A BRIEF HISTORY OF MEDICINE

Since the beginning of time, people have been surviving on this planet by overcoming a variety of conditions and ailments.

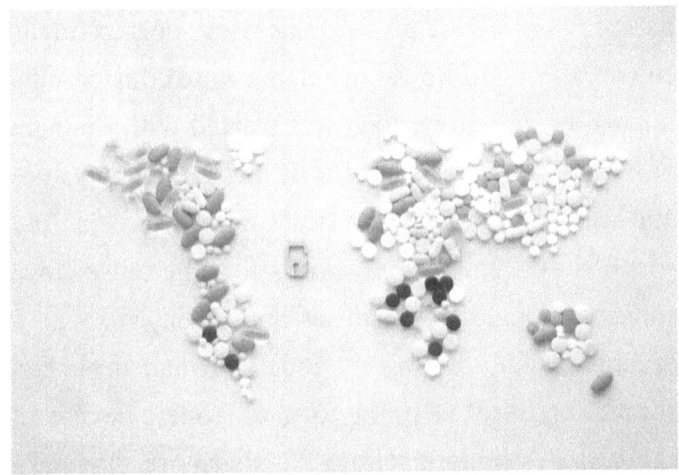

Though pinpointing a particular date to confirm the use of medicine to cure an illness is difficult, it is reasonable to assume that people have discovered a variety of therapeutic options since prehistoric times. With time, however, a progressive advancement in medicine began to emerge, paving the way for a variety of new treatments and approaches to cure diseases.

Medicine Before 1800

History is a vast subject and getting to the root of the origin of medicine can be a daunting task. However, with research over the years, along with evidence from pictorial art and archaeology of primitive surgical tools, there have been different perspectives on death and diseases. For example, constipation and bowel problems were considered a normal occurrence which was treated with the help of herbs. Plants were used for their medicinal values and were researched on a trial-and-error basis. Any sort of severe impairment was said to be caused by a supernatural force, such as an enemy's spell, a demon's curse, or furious gods who had projected something negative in the form of stone or worm in the patient's body and soul. Furthermore, they also utilized counter spells, medicines, suction, and incantations to heal both the body and the soul (Thompson et al., 2020).

According to Thomas (2012), to get the sickness out of the body, a surgical approach of drilling a 2.5 to 5 cm wide hole in the victim's skull was done using a trephine. Trepanning was used in Peru, the United Kingdom, France, and other parts of Europe. This type of procedure is evidenced by the discovery of a few prehistoric trepanned skulls. This practice is still used by a few Indigenous people in Melanesia and Algeria. Throughout the prehistoric age, the use of magic and religion in determining a treatment plan for various ailments was critical. Witch doctors and sorcerers can be considered the first doctors;

they used plant-based medications and a variety of chants and dances to heal their patients. Folk medicines are perhaps the oldest feature of the healing art. Primitive physicians believed in holistic wellness and treated the body and the soul.

Medicine in Ancient Middle East and Egypt

According to Thomas (2012), the dawn of writing marked the onset of recorded history; clay tablets and other forms of records like seals and signs show how physicians in those days carried out their medical practice in ancient Mesopotamia and other regions. For example, the Code of Hammurabi, written by a Babylonian ruler in the 18th century BCE, is preserved on a stone pillar in the Louvre Museum in France. This code provides evidence of how harsh the laws of medical practice were during those days. Failure was punished severely under this code, which included legislation governing the medical profession. For example, if a patient died during treatment, the doctor's hand would be severed, and if the patient was a slave, the doctor would be responsible for finding another slave.

Herodotus, a Greek historian, said that every Babylonian could be considered an amateur physician. The sick would be laid on the street and every passerby could offer their knowledge or advice for the treatment. Divination was extensively used to predict the course of an illness by examining the liver of a sacrificed animal. Unfortunately, not much evidence or information can be found about Babylonian medicine.

Thompson et al. (2020) mentions that the preservation of mummies and the embalming of human bodies reveal a lot about the diseases that were common during the period. Tooth decay, bladder stones, bone tuberculosis, gallstones, gout, arthritis, and parasitic infections were among the ailments. There was no evidence of syphilis or rickets during that period. Further medical research leads to a study of Hebrew literature. Not much information about medicinal practice in Ancient Israel can be found in The Bible, but it does shed light on how Jews were pioneers of personal health and hygiene.

Traditional Medicine in Asia

For many years, India has been known for its

history of medical expertise. Many of the sacred scriptures of the Hindu religion have been solid proof of the medical treatments that have existed for years. Fever, diarrhea, cough, skin problems, tumors, convulsions, and edema were some of the most common health issues treated throughout the Vedic medical period. Though the treatments were cutting-edge, their lack of detailed knowledge of human anatomy slowed them down. The Hindu faith outlawed the cutting of human bodies, which is why this became a worry for the evolution of therapeutic knowledge.

Thompson et al. (2020) suggest that dietetic approaches were primarily used to treat patients, while physicians used the five senses to detect ailments. Inhalations, cupping, and leeching were also used as treatments. It's amazing to think that major surgeries like caesarean sections and amputations were successfully performed back then. The doctors had a lot of experience cutting incisions and removing malignancies. Surgeons used precise punctures to remove toxic fluids from the body, especially the abdomen, in numerous cases. Additionally, many doctors had honed their stitching skills in preparation for the procedures.

China is also noted for its extensive medicinal heritage. The Yellow Emperor wrote *Huangdi neijing*, which was regarded as literature on internal medicine. Only in the early nineteenth century were the Chinese introduced to European medicine. They believed that the human body should have an equal balance of elements: air, wind, water, and fire, so they used them as a strategy to cure ailments. The principle of Yin and Yang was also widely used in body healing at the time.

Mutilation of dead bodies was also highly disregarded in China and because of which, they, very much like the Hindus, had a setback on acquiring knowledge of human anatomy. However, during the year 1798 CE, a major epidemic swept the country and countless lives were lost. It was during this time that a writer of anatomy, Wand Qingren, studied human anatomy with the help of the remains of children that had been torn open by dogs (Thompson et al., 2020).

The Chinese had mastered the art of studying the pulse. They used some of the most effective treatments for a variety of diseases. They employed hydrotherapy, for example, to lower high fevers by giving patients a cool bath. A variety of medicinal herbs were used to relieve pain and heal ailments. Acupuncture is a treatment that is still used today, but it dates back thousands of years.

The Japanese were influenced by Chinese medical methods at the time. Only in the 18th century did medicine begin to show signs of Western influence. It's worth noting that the Japanese were responsible for the discovery of the bacillus plague in 1894, the discovery of the dysentery bacillus in 1897, and the discovery of adrenaline in crystalline form in 1901, which they used in the year 1918 for the first time on cancer that was tar induced.

History of Western Medicine

Early Greece marks the beginning of Western medicine. However, the transition from supernatural and magical beliefs and cures to science, did take a very long time. Greece was known for hundreds of temples and Asclepius was worshipped in those places. Numerous people went to these sites for incubation and temple sleep therapies. The prevalent treatments then were more about diet, exercise, and baths.

Thomas (2012) suggests that by 460 BCE, the year when Hippocrates was born, treatments based on magic were all disregarded. He was later called the father of medicine. He believed in observing the patient in their environment and had a systematic way of diagnosis.

The century that followed Aristotle's work on medicine started to take full ground. He was also called the first biologist. It was his scientific studies that influenced scientific approaches over the next 2,000 years (Thompson et al., 2020).

Medicine During the 19th Century

As you move toward the 19th century, significant aspects that you will notice are the increase in the number of discoveries and also the practice by genuine doctors. By the beginning of this era, the human structure was an open book for medical practitioners. Microscopy and injections had already been invented and were used on a wide scale to treat different conditions. This century became adept with the knowledge of human physiology and germ theory. The discovery entailed the theory that infections were caused due to microscopic living organisms. It was also the age when the first vaccination was used.

The discovery and use of anesthesia was a remarkable achievement in the field of clinical medicine. It was during this century when Thomas Addison gave his name to some blood and adrenal glands disorders. This century did see a burst of eminent personalities who, for centuries, continued to inspire medical practitioners and researchers with their vast knowledge and ideas.

Medicine During the 20th Century

It was this century that brought in some of the best discoveries of treatment that changed many perspectives in the field of medicine. A worth mentioning development in the field of medicine that happened during this century was the study of chemotherapy. There was mass development in every field of medicine: infectious diseases, sulfonamide drugs, antibiotics, penicillin, antituberculosis drugs, immunology, vaccination, endocrinology, insulin, study of sex hormones, vitamins, study of malignant diseases, and surgery procedures, this era saw it all!

After World War II

Warfare does not provide a pleasant sight. It was after World War II that military surgery and many other advanced medical procedures came to the forefront. After the war ended, there were countless injuries and deaths. The doctors and nurses all returned to their normal civilian lives and continued to serve their respective countries by applying their experience of medicine learned on the battlefield for the benefit of others.

Gradually over the years, the development in the field of medicine reached a very high level. From complicated heart surgeries to major organ trans-plant treatments, the medical field has seen the widest range of advancements.

CONTEMPORARY DEMANDS

Change is happening every second, you may not realize the time slipping by, but yes, it is. As we have already touched on, the evolution of medicine and practices took place over the centuries. In recent years too, there have been remarkable advancements in technology and especially in the medical field.

According to The George Washington University School of Business (2020), "The healthcare industry is integral to the physical and 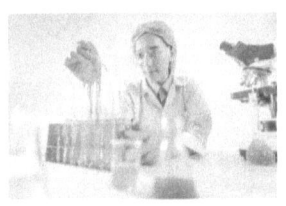 economic health of every person in the U.S. Healthcare professionals are vital to enacting and enforcing policies and keeping the system running efficiently. Today, however, we need these professionals more than ever" (para. 1).

Dr. Mona Hanna-Attisha stated her profound concern about the level of lead in Flint's drinking water in the year 2016. Because of her efforts, she was able to make a significant difference in changing the water sources for drinking water, as lead was posing a significant health risk to children.

There continues to be people, belonging to all different age groups and having numerous health concerns. Due to that issue, combined with changing health policies, the need for a solid healthcare system along with more healthcare professionals is in high demand.

For example, here are a few reasons why there is a great need for more healthcare professionals than ever before.

Aging Baby Boomers

Baby Boomers are referred to those people who were born after the Second World War. The George Washington University School of Business (GW) (2020) reports:

Approximately 76 million people were born between 1946 and 1964, labeled the baby boomer generation, which was the largest in history. The oldest members of this generation reached social security retirement age in 2012; the remaining baby boomers will be of retirement age by 2030. Divide the 76 million baby boomers by the 19-year span of this generation to see an average of four million people retiring annually or nearly 11,000 people per day. (para. 11)

After retirement, the increase of baby boomers relying on Medicaid and Medicare is bound to increase and that can cause problems if there are limited medical resources. A bitter truth is that with the increase in age, there will be an increase in health problems. More facilities and insurance coverage will be required to run the system smoothly and, at the same time, give everyone proper medical access.

With more people reaching a health wise vulnerable age, the pressure of the healthcare department will double. Payment will be a big concern while the treatments are being done. Therefore, it becomes the responsibility of the health departments to keep an eye on the efficient functioning of the insurance systems. The main goal will be to provide the correct medical support to all aging citizens.

More healthcare professionals will be needed as the number of patients surges with time. Not just doctors and nurses, healthcare professionals like other staff, care providers, and professionals to check the IT systems will also be in high demand. People with experience who can add value and the benefit of their experience to the healthcare system should be hired. Expert professionals in technology and leadership should also be utilized as valuable resources ("5 Reasons Why We Need Healthcare Professionals Now More Than Ever," 2020).

Advancement of Technologies

The rapid boom in the advancement of technologies and especially in the medical field has caused several new innovative technologies and ideas to be used for the smooth functioning of the healthcare system. One of the most astounding inventions has been that of home-care monitoring gadgets like the blood glucose and heart rate monitors.

As per the report by GW (2020), "The global home-care diagnostics and monitoring market is predicted to grow 8.71 percent between 2016 and 2020. Technology is the driving force behind the increase" (para. 30).

There are advanced patient monitoring systems from a remote distance and wireless sensor technologies that have made medical practice quite efficient. The doctors and the medical practitioners can observe and guide their patients from any location in the globe. The wireless sensor technology gives comfort to the patients to move around free of any wires that would otherwise hold them back.

With the increase in technologies, there will be a bigger increase in the demand for more healthcare professionals and especially professionals of healthcare informatics. A higher number of people will be required to fill the needed posts that will help make the healthcare system a better place for everyone and most importantly, the patients in need.

Growth of Biopharmaceutical Industry

According to the annual report by Evaluate

Pharma, there has been an increase of 6.3 percent in the rate of growth of the pharmaceutical industry in the year 2022 (as cited in "5 Reasons Why We Need Healthcare Professionals Now More Than Ever," 2020). The demand and supply chain concept works in this case, for instance, with the increase in the number of patients with severe illnesses, there will be the need to produce more drugs and other medical items required for the treatment.

With the increase in the production of biopharmaceutical products, there will be a need for a large number of people who are skilled and educated enough to work for the company. The requirement of medical professionals will be even more. The healthcare system requires professionals who are fast and at the same time highly efficient. People who know chemistry, biology, and clinical research are some of the examples of people who could benefit from getting a job in circumstances like these.

Transformation for the Better

Healthcare is a field that requires a lot of external support as well. Support in the sense of better healthcare policies and advancement of technological aspects. Politics and their different roles in the implementation of various policies have great potential to bring a massive change in society as well as the system. No matter which party forms the government, the main idea is to put together ideas and thoughts of diverse and responsible professionals for the overall development of the medical industry.

Over time, different policies keep on coming to the forefront, but the main point is to understand how well-educated and skilled professionals get opportunities in the healthcare field.

According to GW (2020), "Specialized education is the first step to achieving success in healthcare. Healthcare professionals who want to get involved in the business of healthcare may consider an MBA program that specializes in this industry" (para. 35). However, with every policy and change that will get enforced, there will be a huge requirement of professionals in the healthcare department, especially in the following:

- Healthcare policy jobs: With the recent changes in the healthcare system of the United States, there will be several organizations that will require professionals who have good experience with the health policies. With regards to the policies, these professionals must be able to check if proper protocols are being followed or not.

- Consulting healthcare jobs: Numerous private firms and providers are unable to hire professionals adept with the healthcare policies. These companies get external help from healthcare consulting companies as they have access to the financial modeling and data that is advanced, and which cannot be reached by other organizations.
- Government policy jobs: This is a career that is highly significant as the professionals have an opportunity to influence the policy before its creation. The government employs such healthcare professionals to collect data about the success and failure rate of the ongoing healthcare programs and also asks for suggestions if there are any to help people and the health of the entire community.

When taken a closer look, you will realize how

important a healthcare career can be for you and how it can benefit people in need.

Healthy Competition

Healthy competition is the key to success in any field. If professionals are more enthusiastic about their tasks and career, then there will be healthy growth that can lead to many advantages.

The GW (2020) reports that according to an *Academy of Management Journal* article published in the year 2010, "Competition leads to enhanced creativity when professionals are excited about the task they are performing. When the same people are anxious or nervous about their tasks, competition is more likely to lead to unethical behavior" (para. 24).

A drive to be the best in your career can lead you to find ways that can help you hone your skills even more. For example, according to reports by the Harvard Business School, an increasing number of people are now pursuing an MBA degree to become doctors (as cited in "5 Reasons Why We Need Healthcare Professionals Now More Than Ever," 2020). Similarly, the already experienced doctors are taking up specializations and choosing their desired field more rapidly.

With the rise in awareness about the healthcare system and the careers around it, more people will understand that there are several other options for becoming a medical professional.

WHY IS IT IMPORTANT TO BE PREPARED?

Difficult situations will not be announced before they hit you hard. Especially if the emergency is medical, if you are not prepared, it can lead you to a big problem. Situations may get tense very fast, and if no action is taken immediately, then there will be chances that the situation of concern may rapidly become more serious.

For instance, you may be out in a park with your family or friends and all of a sudden, your friend's finger gets cut open by a sharp tin, but you have no clue as to what action you must take. Now, this can be bad as the cut may lead to severe infection and loss of blood even before the medics arrive.

However, if you've had your share of knowledge about medical emergencies, then you'd know what to do immediately to stop the excess blood flow. The first step that you would do is clean the wound with some water and apply pressure on the finger to keep it intact and also to stop bleeding. By the time medics arrived, you would have taken good care of the situation.

Therefore, you can see how even in the simplest of situations, your preparedness with medical knowledge can help lessen someone's pain and more so, even save lives.

BECOMING A MEDICAL ASSET

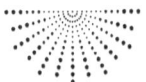

*F*rom the dawn of civilizations to modern times, one thing that has always been the most beneficial for every living being on earth is medical care and preparedness. As you already know by now, even the tiniest of health issues can cause severe threats to lives. Negligence and a laid-back attitude toward health can cause serious harm in the long run. The truth is, you have people you care about all around you, like your friends, family, and loved ones. Just the thought of any of them, including you, falling victim to some kind of health emergency can be nerve-racking in itself. The truth is also that if medical care is given to anyone at the right time, a huge problem can be lessened or even prevented.

However, as an individual who understands the importance of grave circumstances and the benefit of the medical 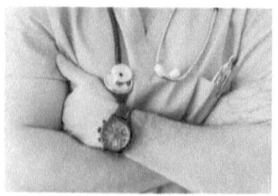 system, you must first ensure yourself that you can be prepared and help others, especially when you are on an expedition to outdoor terrains. One of the first steps that you must take before going to the wilderness is to understand every member's fitness level: if they have any pre-existing health conditions like cardiac issues, breathing issues like asthma, allergies, etc. Another important factor that you must check is if the weather is suitable. Having clear knowledge of the upcoming weather forecasts is mandatory. Last but not the least, you must be prepared, and so should you prepare your fellow companions as to how to handle the situation if anyone gets hurt during the adventure. After all, if it's you that is injured, having given some prior knowledge to your group, might very well allow them to properly help you.

BASIC MEDICAL EDUCATION

Once you've made up your mind to become a medical asset, you need to understand what medical knowledge that you must learn.

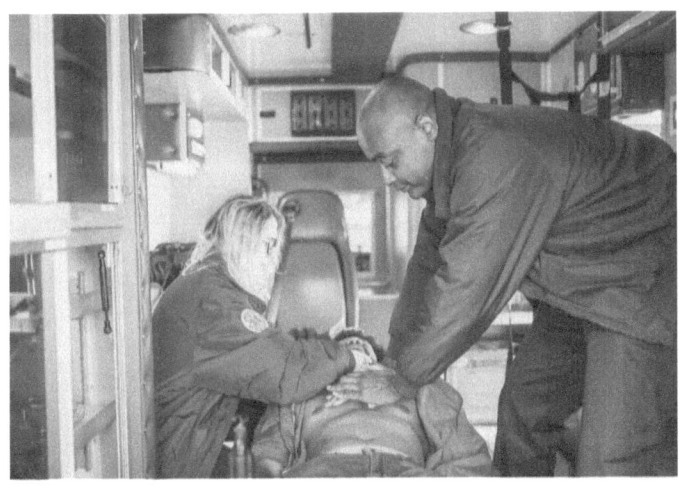

Cardiopulmonary Resuscitation (CPR)

CPR is a life-saving emergency procedure. It requires a series of chest compressions along with artificial ventilation. The main purpose of this method is to keep brain function, breathing, and blood circulation in place until medical help arrives. It is an easy-to-learn process and can be beneficial in a huge way.

Set a Splint

This is a method of setting up a stabilizing mechanism in an emergency to help a broken arm or leg stay in place. During an emergency, it can be made of any available sticks and clothes. This process helps the bones to remain intact and prevent excess pain that can be caused by movements. This is a highly recommended method that could be used if someone in your group ends up breaking their bones. You may be in the wilderness, far from help, but this technique can keep the fractured and broken bone at rest for some time.

Burn Treatment

Treatment of burns can be tricky as there are three different degrees of burns. When a person gets burned, you will have to determine the burn level. For example, if it is just a first-degree burn, then make sure to apply a soothing ointment on the affected areas and cover it with a thin gauge. If the burn has resulted in some blisters and has created a bit of swelling, then that can be termed as a second-degree burn. In this case, you will have to run it under cold water and apply an ointment over it.

However, the third-degree is the most acute of all and will require the immediate help of a doctor.

Spot a Concussion

A concussion can occur as a result of a blow to the head caused by a hit or fall. Particularly in the outdoors, you must be able to determine whether or not someone has suffered a concussion. Examine the pupil to check whether it has dilated and ask the patient if they are dizzy or experiencing any discomfort. If a serious concussion is not treated promptly, it might cause permanent brain damage.

Heimlich Maneuver

Choking is hazardous, especially if proper first aid is not provided. The Heimlich Maneuver is a technique for helping a choking person push out whatever was restricting their airways by giving an abdominal thrust above the naval area. You should fist your hands and press into the upper naval area back and forth until the impediment is gone. You can perform this maneuver on yourself by using a hard, solid, stationary item (chair, counter, log, rock, etc.) and pressing your body forcibly against it.

Stop the Bleeding

This is one of the topmost medical aids that you must be aware of. A person could excessively bleed and lose their life quite quickly. You must know how to make a tourniquet to combat rapid blood loss.

By following some of these important first aid techniques you will be able to save your own life as well as the lives of many others.

WILDERNESS BASIC MEDICAL EDUCATION

One of the primary motivations for embarking on a journey into the wilderness is to immerse oneself in nature while remaining as remote as possible from the hustle and bustle of cities and towns. I'm sure there aren't many things that can provide the same level of tranquility as the wilderness. Several people yearn for serenity as well as a profound desire to enjoy the outdoors while also feeding their curiosity about wildlife.

The farther you travel into the wilderness, the farther you will be from any medical facility or emergency department. Staying outdoors has many advantages, but one of the most severe disadvantages is the difficulty in seeking medical treatment.

As you travel through the deepest reaches of the mountains and forests, the chances are very high that you will be bitten by a swarm of insects and may even come face-to-face with an animal or two. Tents can be tough to live in, and the weather can be harsh at times. In such a situation, just imagine someone on your team facing some major health issue; the probability will be high that they will suffer, but if you have adept knowledge about how to deal with medical issues, then that can be a great advantage.

Your Immediate Actions

There are many aspects that you'll have to be careful about while going out in the wilderness alone or with a group. However, if you have even the slightest suspicion that something is going wrong, and the nearest emergency services are a long way away, a few first aid basics should be added to your other important first aid actions (Schimelpfenig, 2020):

- Try to evaluate the person who is in pain.
- Understand the scene.
- Identify what could be life-threatening.

- Ask for the patient's medical history.
- Conduct a head-to-toe exam and look for any threatening signs and symptoms.
- Check the eyes for signs of a concussion.
- Immediately start thinking about what the medical care plan should be for the patient.
- Prepare for immediate evacuation in case the medical relief people arrive.
- Continuously make an effort to check the condition of the patient.

These are some of the most important steps that you can follow to ensure that the patient is safe and conscious.

First Aid in the Wilderness Can Be Tricky

When considering first aid in the wilderness, keep in mind that it will be considerably different from what you would do in a city or town with medical services nearby. Here are some of the factors that influence wilderness treatment:

- When you witness someone suffering or being harmed, the first thing that comes to mind is to call 911! That's not going to work in the woods. The terrain is difficult, and the woodlands are dense, so getting medical help will be next to impossible. As a result, if you find yourself in the middle of a medical emergency while backpacking, you must be prepared to care for the patient and keep them safe for a long time, at least until a medical rescue team arrives. It could take days, weeks, or even months at times. Therefore, it is up to you to take all the necessary first aid actions.

- To stay prepared in the event of a medical emergency in the wild, have the most important medicines and equipment with you at all costs. Carry your medical gear with you at all times and be prepared to treat a patient with whatever supplies you have on hand. For example, at a hospital, when a patient who is dehydrated and has diarrhea, they are given IV fluid therapy. In the wild, though, the situation will be different. If you don't have access to an IV, you'll need to give the patient plenty of water. You might also use electrolyte powders or salt and sugar water instead.

- In the outdoors, communication can be the most difficult. Without a doubt, technological and network coverage have improved in many challenging regions, but owing to network unavailability or fluctuating coverage, even sending a text message, deep in the woods could take a long time. As a result, if you're in the middle of nowhere and have a medical emergency, things might get complicated quickly because though you'll be carrying your cell phone, you could find it extremely difficult to call people for help.

- When you're out in the woods, the weather may have a big impact. Though various weather forecast applications clearly show you the approaching weather of a location ahead of time, you can still be subjected to many untold complications caused by sudden changes in the air. You will have to make it in tents and eat and drink the few supplies that you've carried. Therefore, if at night you get very chilly, you will have no option like a bigger blanket to ease you. All that you will be able to do is light a fire and drink some hot tea to keep yourself warm.

Therefore, if you've decided to have an adventure-filled life in the wild, then these are some of the things that you must be aware of and should be ready to live with.

Protocols to Follow While Giving Treatment in the Wilderness

The treatment process of a patient in the wilderness can be quite different from that in a medical room. A few vital methods of treatment procedures and a few protocols that you can follow before and while treating a patient are listed below as guidance (Schimelpfenig, 2020):

- Always check the area where the patient fell sick or got injured. There might be clues as to what could have caused the injury or health hazard. For example, take a look around to see if there are any traces of poisonous creatures or plants that could have caused an adverse reaction. Also, if the patient gets hit by something or is found in a slippery or high place, make sure to take them to a safe and clean area.

- Look for others who have been injured, too. There might be people who assume they are fine and could even look fine, but in reality, they could be suffering from trauma or concussion.

- Always ask for consent to go ahead with the treatment—if the patient is in a conscious state.

- If the patient is unconscious, make an effort to bring them back to consciousness.

- Treat every unknown disease as infectious. Always wear a mask, and a pair of gloves to keep yourself protected at all times.

- Check how serious the injury or illness is and accordingly, devise a plan to start the medical procedure.

Having followed the above protocols, you can perform the following essential first aid actions following the ABCDE rule (Schimelpfenig, 2020):

- A: Always check the airway. Examine the

entire mouth to see if there are any obstructions.

- B: Go near the chest and check if the patient is breathing normally or not.
- C: Ensure to check the patient's pulse and also look around if there are any signs of internal or external bleeding.
- D: If the patient hurts the spine, there will be chances of a temporary disability. Protect the spine area in case you cannot find the cause of the immobility.
- E: Exposure of injuries is a must, open the tight clothes of the patient and check if there are any injuries.

As a result, by checking various indicators of the patient, such as heart rate and peculiar odors, as well as excessive bleeding and signs of the skin turning pale or blue, you will be able to understand the reasons for health problems and, as a result, be able to treat them on time, even in the wild.

TOP TIPS FOR WILDERNESS MEDICAL EMERGENCIES

As an outdoor enthusiast, I've had my fair share of emergencies. There have been numerous incidents while trekking through snow-capped regions to dry forest areas that have taught me how to deal with medical issues in the wild. However, here are some of the most prevalent medical hazards that can occur outdoors at any moment.

The truth is that there is not as significant of a difference as you might think between the medication used in the wild and that used in health facilities. Similarly, patient behavior does not depend on location. The patient's personality has a role in dealing with medical issues, whether they are outdoors or confined to a hospital room, since some people get terrified at the sight of a drop of blood, while others may treat even a major cut not so seriously. In both circumstances, treating such people can be dangerous.

However, the setting may be so bizarre that stabilizing a tough medical emergency in the wild will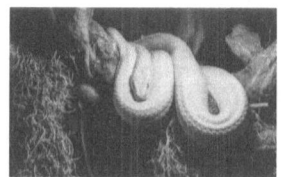

require a lot of focus and tenacity.

According to Decker (2018), here are some tips that could help save lives in the wilderness:

- Snake bite: If a snake bites you, immediately try to take a picture of the snake to figure out the venom type. Wash the bite area and bandage it. Never try to suck the venom out. Immediately rush the patient to the hospital for antivenom treatment.
- Hypothermia: If someone is hypothermic, ensure that the person is wrapped up with a space blanket or a foil. Provide warm compress throughout the body of the patient. If the condition persists, you can use the technique of your body heat treatment. Give the patient frequent hot water or tea.
- Open scalp wound: In case of a major accident and the scalp opens wide, until the medical rescue team arrives, you can tie the hair of the patient across the wound to keep it in a stable position.
- Insect bites: Always use an insect repellant when you are outdoors. However, use

Plantago (plantain) to help soothe the irritation. It can also be helpful for sunburns.

- Diabetics: Always carry honey to treat low blood sugar. At times when people start hiking, they tend to forget to eat on time and prolonged aerobic exercise lowers blood sugar. Honey is a great way to raise glucose levels and can be rubbed on the gums if the person is unresponsive. Honey is also said to be a great antibiotic.

- Check dehydration correctly: Hyponatremia is a condition in which the body's sodium level goes below normal. Hyponatremia affects a large number of people. This has been observed during expeditions through the Grand Canyon, where people mistakenly believe they are dehydrated and drink large amounts of water (Myers & Hoffman, 2015). As a result, you should always check the color of your urine to see if it is overly concentrated (the darker the urine, the more dehydrated you are). If a person is dehydrated, provide them with not only water but also sufficient nutrition.

- Injured bone: When you encounter a situation where a patient has probably broken or fractured some part of their body. Then, make sure you immobilize them. Make use of any stick or rods that are available nearby to give support to the affected part.

- Purify water: In the wilderness, the best way to purify water is to boil it. Make sure that you boil for a little longer than the boiling point to ensure that all harmful bacteria is killed in the process.

- Use feminine hygiene products: Products like sanitary pads can be of great help while out in the wild. They can be used to give padding to an injury or to help seal a wound. Tampons on the other hand are perfect to stop nose bleeds.

- Carry a headlamp: This should be on the priority list of the accessories needed for a wild expedition. The nights can be very dark and with many things to carry and do, a headlamp can free your hands and be extremely easy to use.

- Altitude sickness: This can be a serious issue for someone who faces challenges in

high-altitude regions. The first step for
you would be to make the patient descend
to a lower altitude region.

We have discussed a large number of possible medical emergencies and the ways to overcome them all. However, the point is, there are important accessories that you should always have by your side while on an expedition in the wild. A few of the most essential tools that will be of great help to you in the wilderness as mentioned by Buer (2016) include:

- safety pins
- trauma shears
- wilderness guidebook
- thermometer
- antibiotic ointments
- 2nd skin dressings
- bandages
- sam splint
- gloves
- antiseptic towels
- povidone-iodine solutions
- wound closure strips
- cotton swabs

- tweezers
- scissors
- band-aids
- 12cc irrigation syringe
- 1-inch cloth tape
- sterile scrub brush
- 4-6 inch elastic wrap
- 4x4 sterile gauze pads

With the correct tools in place, any health problem can be given good medical support.

KNOW YOUR SURROUNDINGS

Your confidence is what will enable you to conquer even the most difficult conditions in your life. When you're on a wilderness adventure and you're going to new places, you should always make sure you know what the landscape is like and the methods to deal with situations related to it.

HEAT

According to a report by Lipman et at. (2014), in the last decade, more than 600 people succumbed to death due to causes related to excessive exposure to heat. Heat-related illnesses are very common, and many people suffer due to them. It is a condition in which the body temperature of a person reaches a very high level resulting in organ damage, including the brain, kidney, heart, and even muscles. Some of the heat-related issues are hyperthermia, heat cramps, heat exhaustion, heatstroke, and heat syncope. Few drugs and medications are also considered to be a big cause for heat-related illnesses such as antipsychotics, antihistamines, alcohol, amphetamines, alpha-adrenergic, beta-blockers, benzodiazepines, calcium-channel blockers, cocaine, clopidogrel, diuretics, laxatives, phenothiazines, thyroid agonists, tricyclic antidepressants, and neuroleptics.

In their article, Lipman et al. (2014) provide some of the ways to reduce the body temperature of patients:

- One of the most common ways to reduce the body heat of a person is to take them to a shaded area that has access to cool air. Most suitably if the room or the place is below the temperature of 20°C (68°F).
- Hydration is the key to curing water deficiencies and can substantially reduce

hyperthermia. However, ensure that the patient does not get overhydrated as that will cause pulmonary edema.

- Immersion in cold water can be a very effective way of reducing body temperature. It can substantially prevent heat stroke.
- Evaporative cooling is another measure by which heat of the body can be reduced if no immersion facility is available. This is done by loosening the clothes of the patient and sprinkling cold water onto the body to reduce body heat.
- Ice packs and chemical packs are some of the most convenient ways to reduce body heat. You can apply them externally to the skin in the neck and groin regions to reduce excessive heat.
- Ice towel application is another very simple way to help reduce body heat.
- Antipyretics are used to treat elevated temperatures.

There are innumerable ways to counter illnesses caused by excessive body heat, and one of the best ways is by making the body cool down using natural methods that are easily accessible.

COLD

Issues like hypothermia, frostbite, and many other injuries are problems that affect people who venture out in the wilderness during excessively cold weather. Cold weather can harm the health of some people even if they do not go outdoors.

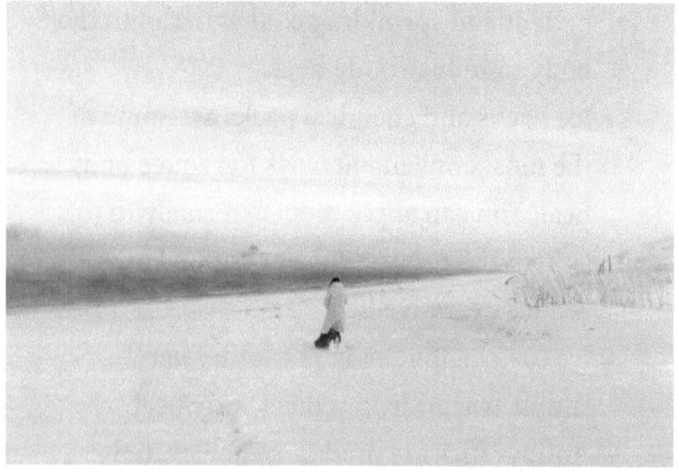

Different individuals will have different levels of endurance to cold. Hypothermia is a condition in which the body temperature falls below 35°C (95°F). Some of the common symptoms of hypothermia are exhaustion, extreme shivering, feeble memory, slurred speech, fumbling hands, drowsiness, and lack of coordination.

Hypothermia, if left untreated, can result in heart and breathing system failure, as well as death. A person with hypothermia usually is not aware of their condition right at the beginning. Due to this reason, people may become perplexed in their behavior as a result of this illness.

If you face a situation where someone is suffering through this condition, you should take the following action ("Hypothermia," 2020):

- Handle the patient with extra gentleness. Do not massage or rub the patient as vigorous movement can cause cardiac arrest.
- Immediately take the patient to a warmer place. However, if moving is not possible, then keep the patient in a horizontal position and cover with warm blankets.
- Remove wet clothes immediately.
- Cover the patient with warm clothes and blankets.
- Monitor heart rate and breathing continuously and if by any chance you

realize that there is no pulse, then immediately start with CPR.

- Use a warm compress to increase the body temperature of the patient. Apply the warm compress on the chest, neck, and groin. Refrain from applying a compress to the feet and arms because doing so can cause the cold blood to circulate back to the brain, lungs, and heart. This can cause a serious drop in the body temperature and that could be dangerous.

- Give warm beverages to the patient, but only do so if the patient is conscious.

- Do not use hot water bags or heating pads directly to the patient's skin because that may suddenly heat the body and could cause irregular heartbeat.

Therefore, be careful next time when you deal with someone suffering from hypothermia.

Frostbite is another severe problem that people face while exposed to extremely low temperatures. When the skin and underlying tissue get injured due to the cold and the damage is not very permanent, then that condition is called frostnip. This condition can be treated with the help of warming the affected areas. However, if the condition is severe, then it is frostbite.

Numbness, waxy-looking hard skin, muscle stiffness, prickling feeling, reddish or bluish skin, and blistering can emerge when rewarmed. These are some of the key indications and symptoms of frostbite. If the swelling and agony worsen, as well as if you develop a fever, you should see a doctor immediately ("Frostbite," 2021).

According to the Mayo Clinic (2021), until the medical team arrives you can attend to the condition of frostbite by following a few measures:

- Remove wet clothes from the body.
- Cover all the affected areas and keep them safe from the cold wind and air.
- Do not walk if you have frostbite on your legs.
- Do not try to roughly move the parts of your body affected by frostbite.
- You can use a painkiller to help deal with the agony caused.

ADAPT TO ALTITUDE

Without visiting a region with steep terrain and greater altitude, treks and hikes just feel incomplete to those of us who love an outdoor adventure. Most people who enjoy the concept of discovering new locations and nature must have felt the need to adjust to the altitude at some point in their lives. However, as beautiful as the higher terrains can be, some people can face equally bigger health issues due to high altitude.

High altitude illnesses are common and there are some very effective ways to prevent such symptoms. There has been a surge of traveling to higher peaks in recent years. For instance, a UK-based company offered around 93 expeditions to Mount Kilimanjaro in just 12 months. However, with the increase in such expeditions, the chances of more people falling sick due to high altitude will also escalate. Similarly, cases from the Rocky Mountains and European Alps have reported similar illnesses all caused due to altitude (Shah et al., 2015).

While hiking on a steep slope or toward a higher altitude, many times you may not realize whether it is just the normal panting that is happening due to the climb uphill or whether you are having a breathing issue. In such a case, always note a few key signs and symptoms ("Altitude Sickness," 2020):

- headache
- dizziness
- nausea
- vomiting
- inability to walk
- coordination problem
- feeling of suffocation
- persistent cough
- disorientation
- chest congestion
- fatigue
- breathlessness

Once you've identified any of such signs in yourself or anyone around you, make sure to take the following steps ("Altitude Sickness," 2020):

- Every sickness that is related to shortness of breath, nausea, vomiting, and headaches should be considered to be altitude sickness until proven otherwise. If these signs persist, immediately stop the climb and descend to a lower altitude.

- While going on a hike uphill, always follow the graded ascent rule; do not over climb in one day.
- If any of the people with you feel any discomfort, address their issue immediately; do not wait for their condition to worsen.
- Keep an eye on the patient.
- Generally, within 1-2 days most patients start recovering. However, be extra alert.
- For headaches, you can administer Ibuprofen and acetaminophen (Tylenol). Always be careful about the correct and safe dosage.
- Do not allow the patient to have any sleeping pills.

Climbing uphill can be a stressful task under normal conditions, but when the harsh climate of the hilly areas is added on, then there can be more stress. Due to such exertion, you may experience discomfort and some signs of illness. Take any sign seriously and stop hiking immediately if you feel any kind of discomfort in your health.

NATURAL DISASTERS

Natural disasters are reported to cause roughly 500 deaths each year in the United States alone (Cormier, 2017). In the sphere of disaster management, disaster preparedness and healthcare resources frequently fall short. Staff members in the hospital, family members of patients, and, most crucially, the patient in question, are all at risk in the event of such a situation.

Anyone can become a victim of a natural disaster, no matter how much people plan as per weather reports and other forecasts; the fact is that elements of nature work in their bizarre way and sometimes can be very unpredictable.

When a natural disaster strikes, no one is spared. Therefore, the most important point is that there should be adept planning and preparation for any case that is related to a natural disaster. Here are a few tips by which there can be a more planned approach toward managing a natural disaster situation:

Communication

Problems that people face as a result of organization-wide actions and policies can be solved with clear communication. Many times in the past, organizations have hesitated to provide precise information to the public. This approach is disadvantageous since it can lead to a slew of misunderstandings and, more importantly, plenty of unfounded speculations. There will be widespread panic, especially after catastrophic events, but this can be alleviated and calmed to a large extent if healthcare services make an effort to explain the situation to the public. People will respond positively to information provided by a healthcare authority.

Even within the organization, there should be clear-cut communication between the members and staff. Everyone should be informed about the ongoing situation. Effective implementation of protocols and plans can be done only by having everyone on the same page. Every top-tier department, including management and government affiliates, should be aware of the current state of affairs.

Training

When a natural disaster strikes, the healthcare system should be more prepared than any other department, as there will be a risk of numerous people getting injured. Just because a flood has not happened in the last two decades does not mean that it will not hit any time soon. Preparation is key, and training is the only way in which a huge part of the situation can be handled in times of crisis.

A laid-back attitude by organizations and their employees can be harmful as one will never know when an emergency can hit a place. Therefore, all the healthcare staff should be given intensive training to understand how to manage things during times of natural crisis. Healthcare organizations should conduct emergency preparedness drills, coordinating with local emergency response agencies and the public whenever possible.

Technological Protocols

Hospital management and employees have discovered that access to patient data and hospital documents becomes inaccessible after a natural calamity, causing considerable damage to the hospital's property as well.

Not only should the tangible room where important and valuable documents are kept be improved, but the data stored in various files should also be stored appropriately to save important information.

Healthcare Leadership

Hospitals and other medical facilities are so preoccupied with their day-to-day tasks of treating innumerable patients that the healthcare administration staff frequently overlook outdated catastrophe plans. Medical facilities, for example, should be self-sufficient to give quality medical care and emergency treatment to persons injured or traumatized, even in the event of a disaster. This way, they may gain the trust of the community while also serving them, which will be extremely advantageous to their ability to generate more revenue from the service.

The essential point is that hospitals deal with difficult situations and emergencies regularly, but all higher authorities should keep natural disasters and protocols for dealing with them as a top priority as well. If there are any approaching disasters, every department must be well versed in their preparations. They should constantly be prepared to meet any crisis with tenacity and efficiency.

Knowledge of Assets

Hospital authorities must be prepared for emergencies of all kinds of natural disasters as well.

When a natural disaster occurs, it becomes a horrendous task for the government officials and hospital authorities to attend to every single person affected or hurt. There will be a massive rush in the hospital that may make it impossible to rely on any outside help. Keeping in mind such situations, it is imperative for healthcare organizations, especially hospitals, to be aware of the supplies and assets that they have.

MAJOR EVENTS

Major events are disasters, causing unimaginable destruction to the people, community, and environment. Some examples of events with prolonged risk of threat include radiological, biological, and chemical disasters.

Radiation

History has seen some of the cruelest and painful radiation disasters. The majority of these have been caused by severe nuclear power plant explosions, which were primarily triggered by accidents. Whatever the origin, the consequences of such incidents have resulted in damage that is beyond repair. For example, the Windscale Fire Nuclear Disaster in the United Kingdom in 1957, the Three Mile Island Nuclear Accident in Pennsylvania, USA in 1979, and the 2011 Fukushima Nuclear Disaster in Japan ("The Five Worst Nuclear Disasters in History," 2014).

Aside from major catastrophes, it is also a reality that radiation exists in the form of background radiation, which is produced by natural minerals.

Kim (2018) asserts that "for reducing radiation exposure, there are three principals: time, distance, and shielding" (para. 1). 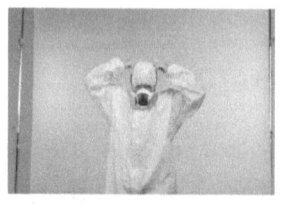 However, in the event of a calamity caused by an accident or even a terrorist strike, there are a few steps you can take to keep yourself safe:

- Understanding the three aspects of time, distance, and shielding can be very useful.
- Under unavoidable situations, limiting the time of radiation exposure can be a good way to minimize the effect of radiation.
- Maintaining a distance from the source of radiation can help in reducing the effect.
- Creating a barrier of lead, water, or

concrete can minimize the penetration of x-rays and gamma rays drastically.

- In case of a sudden radiation emergency, stay indoors (a concrete building is best), and close all the openings like windows and doors.
- Stay in the sheltering place until and unless the authorities pass on information to get a contamination screening done.

Radiation exposure can cause serious health hazards like radiation sickness, skin burns, heart issues, and also cancer. Therefore, whenever there is a chance of you getting exposed to any place or object that could be contaminated with radiation, ensure that you follow strict measures and keep yourself and others around you safe and sound.

Biological

Biological hazards can cause major life risks to humans and animals. Toxin, microorganisms, spores, fungi, and viruses are some of the examples of such substances. Biohazards can affect any environment and include pathological waste, human body fluids, animal byproducts, sharps, infectious waste, human blood, and recombinant DNA and RNA. Here are a few best practice methods that you could follow to stay safe in an environment plagued with biohazards (Burns, 2009):

- Universal precaution: Treat every situation with grave concern. Deal with every potential biohazard like blood or any other infectious item as dangerous.
- Gloves: Clean your hands and check if the gloves are in good condition. Check for leakages or anything inside that could harm your health. Thoroughly clean your hands and then wear your gloves. Do not touch anything with bare hands, and when you are done, carefully dispose of the gloves in a safe biohazard bin.
- Body protection: In cases of extreme contamination, ensure that you have personal protective equipment (PPE) like a proper body jacket, apron, or other suit ready. Ensure you wear them at all times and discard them well after you are done.
- Face protection: Ensure you always use eye goggles, a face mask, and most importantly a face shield at all times.

- Clean-Up: Cleaning up is a process that is vital for decontaminating an area. Always carry a biohazard bag and kit in situations where you will need to do a lot of clean-up. Put on your gloves and protection gear while going through the process. Use disinfectants and sometimes a bit of bleach to clean places that have been contaminated.
- Sanitize the equipment: Clean the space thoroughly and then use a professional person to sanitize the area and the equipment that cannot be discarded.
- Decontamination: After you've done your work, clean your hands with antiseptic wipes and let them air dry. Go to a washroom and wash your hands and the parts of your body that have been potentially exposed with a strong soap.

There has been an increase in the improper disposal of trash products in recent years. If those who work with biohazards are not attentive in classifying waste products as biohazards, it may generate problems for those who work in the cleaning department. Keep an eye out for sharp edges that could be contaminated. Make sure you break them down safely and dispose of them in biohazard garbage bags.

Infections relating to biohazards can be dangerous. However, by understanding the risks involved and by spreading awareness, a lot can be brought under control.

Chemical

Chemicals can be dangerous if they are not handled with care and extreme caution. Substances that are non-biological that can pose threat to human and animal life are chemical hazards. Unfortunately, chemicals have become a big part of our daily lives. These days, there is a presence of chemicals in a majority of things. From the food that we eat to the cleaning agents that we use in our homes, all contain some chemicals.

There are three main ways in which you may come in contact with chemical hazards: food and water, air, and touching a potential chemical hazard. Here are a few ways by which chemical hazards can be prevented by following a few measures:

- Prevent chemical accidents by being extra

cautious, avoiding mixing of chemicals, and storing the chemicals in a place accessible to only authorized personnel.

- Prevent fire accidents caused by chemicals by keeping them in a fireproof storeroom.
- Prevent spillage by being very careful. If there are any spills, make sure to get it cleaned thoroughly by following the right measures.
- Dispose of unused chemicals carefully. Do not throw them in places that could be dangerous to the water supply and wildlife, too.
- If you find someone is poisoned, immediately call the poison control authorities.

In the event of a chemical hazard accident, do not panic! Read and follow the instructions given by the authorities and follow every single step as mentioned. Follow the news and radio and stay sheltered until they declare the situation is under control.

With the wealth of information available on healthcare facilities and how to become a medical asset, it's clear why medical knowledge is so important for survival. Whether you believe in living in the wilderness like me or not, there is always the possibility that anything could go wrong in your everyday life. The guidance that is provided in this chapter can be helpful in unforeseen times. You may be out in the wild and by knowing how to tackle every situation, you will be confident to take any journey without a hiccup. The confidence that you get as a result of being knowledgeable is something that you cannot compare with any other knowledge. It is the thought that you know your loved ones and the people around you are safe that gives a great sense of life satisfaction. As a result, comprehending problems and generating strategies to get out of them can be a huge accomplishment. You can save the lives of many people by educating yourself as a medical asset.

3

THE POWER OF NATURAL MEDICINE

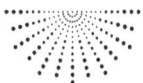

The enigma around planet earth and its rich composition of plants and living organisms will always remain a beauty. Throughout the ages, humans and animals have survived some of the toughest challenges that civilizations face. Natural calamities like floods, droughts, landslides, volcanic eruptions, and at times even meteors, have ravaged many parts of the world. Epidemics and pandemics have been very prevalent over the course of evolution.

With time, there has been massive development in the field of medicine and technology. No matter to what level the allopathic

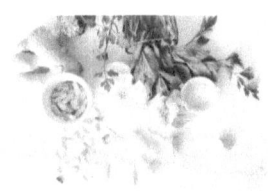

range of medicine and its treatments have reached, the importance of natural medicine cannot be over-looked. If you think about it, how have people and animals been surviving numerous illnesses since the beginning of time and also before the discovery of modern medicine? This proves the point that there is a plethora of natural herbs and remedies that have the power to solve and cure many diseases and ailments. The health benefits that can be found in natural products and the medicines created from natural plants and other sources can be said to be humongous.

You must be confused as to how plants and herbs that you hardly know the names of can be used for medicinal purposes. If you are out in the wild, you may not be equipped with the best medicines all the time; it is in a scenario like this that nature and natural medicine can save your life. By acquiring correct knowledge about natural medicines, you will know what to do next time you need some relief.

NATURAL MEDICINE IS THE WAY!

The modern world is exposed to the dangers of chemicals and pollution. At times like this, contamination of any sort can cause serious life-threatening problems. The healthcare industry has regularly seen a huge influx of patients suffering from new and different types of diseases. There are many cases where allopathic medicines can prove to be too strong to the body and mind; they may heal you but can at the same time have the potential to cause innate harm if not taken in the correct dosages. However, there is a reduced chance of adverse effects with natural medicines.

Natural medicine follows the principles of self-healing and vitalism techniques. A naturopathic doctor will almost always ask you to not get parallel treatment for the same condition from an allopathic doctor. The reason why contemporary medicines and other medical procedures are encouraged to be avoided is that they believe that the body takes its due course of time to heal and is capable of self-healing provided the right methods are used ("Naturopathy," 2021).

It may take a while for the person who has always been exposed to allopathic treatments to understand the benefits of natural medicines. This makes it essential for you to understand the details of natural medicines and their benefits to help guide others who are in need of natural based care.

Benefits of Natural Medicines

Apart from the systematic and holistic healing process used to balance out the entire system, including body and mind, there are other essential reasons why opting for natural medicines would be a good decision. The Institute for Natural Medicine (n.d.) discusses the need for and some of the benefits of using naturopathy:

- More affordable: Healthcare costs in the United States have been on a rise for quite some time. At such a time, policymakers have been urging medical practitioners from various fields including naturopathic doctors and primary care doctors to play their roles in making an effort to provide valuable service to the people in terms of their health and well-being. The main priority of the healthcare system should be to look into the health of people apart from just providing the treatments.
- Not just the policy-related matters, it has been seen that natural treatment has a wide range of options that can be way less in cost than in comparison to

conventional methods. Naturopathic treatments believe in curing the root cause, therefore, the cost for medicines and surgeries focused on treating just the symptoms can be greatly reduced. Healthcare and insurance costs that are often used for the treatment of cases resulting from adverse reactions of conventional medicines are also substantially reduced.

- Reduced side effects: Natural treatments are said to cause zero to a minimal level of side effects. Natural medicines are made from herbs and everything that is of nature. There are no harmful chemicals involved because patients usually do not experience any adverse reactions from their usage.

- Health promotion: At times when the conventional method of treatment and medication seems to fail, numerous people start looking for alternative medicine. It is in such a situation when natural medicines enter the scene. Natural medicines are said to be non-toxic and safe which makes it one of the most desired methods of treatment. Natural techniques of healing are a great means of treating pain. Hence, a holistic approach to treating pain is often adopted.

- Easier to obtain than prescription medicine: Requiring a prescription to acquire medication can be expensive, tedious, and difficult, demanding doctor visits, regular tests, and continual efforts with refills and insurance. In comparison, natural medicines are easily available and do not cost as much.

- Natural healing: Natural medication is all about treating the entire mind and body together as one. This technique makes an effort to find the underlying cause of any health condition. The practitioners of this method think that the body has the potential to self-heal. With much time given, natural medicines can show their effect in curing a person for better health.

- Strengthen the immune system: There are numerous herbs and natural items that are beneficial to strengthening the immune system. It is your immune system that protects you from any form of illness that enters your body and fights harmful health threats. Some of the herbs and medicines that are natural are said to boost energy and at the same time, increase the efficiency of your immune system.

- Naturopathic medicines are available for any age: In conventional methods of treatment, many medicines are prescribed with keeping in mind the age of a person. People suffering from exhaustion, stress, and other related disorders are most likely to opt for a treatment that can have no side effects in the long run. People of any age can opt for a natural medicinal treatment that cannot just cure their sickness, but can at the same time cause no damage to their organs.

What Are Herbal Medicines?

Herbal medicine is the application of plants and herbs to make medications by integrating their therapeutic properties, scent, and even taste. A majority of people turn to herbal medications from conventional treatments in order to gain better health benefits and improve their holistic well-being. Teas, fresh plants, dried plants, plant extracts, pills, and capsules are all commonly used forms of herbal medicine.

There is a widespread fallacy that all medicines labelled as 'natural' are entirely safe for wellness. This isn't always the case, though. One concern with herbal medicines is that they are not subjected to the same rigorous standards of testing and trial practices as conventional approaches.

A few herbs, such as ephedra and comfrey, are thought to be hazardous if used incorrectly. As a result, you should strive to seek a trustworthy recommendation from a natural doctor, and also inform your health practitioner before testing any of these plants as medicines.

What Are Naturopathic Medicines?

Natural medicine refers to the natural remedies that are used to cure and heal the body. There are quite a few different types of naturopathic therapies that include acupuncture, exercise, massage, natural counseling, and most important of all, herbs. The United States was introduced to naturopathic medicine in the 1800s. However, it cannot be denied that some of the treatment procedures are derived from age-old practices and knowledge.

It is considered that naturopathy belongs to the era of 400 BC, and it was Hippocrates, a Greek philosopher, who ciphered the principles of the practice. The practice of natural medicine is considered to be a wide range of pseudoscientific methods and is often termed natural, self-healing, and non-invasive. The practitioners of natural medication are referred to as naturopathic doctors and they have to undergo professional qualifications and obtain required licenses to practice their medical knowledge ("What is Natural Medicine," 2021).

There are numerous kinds of practitioners specializing in their respective fields and because of which, generalizing them into one particular type is a difficult task. The treatments done via natural methods can range from homeopathy, open quackery, and also to psychotherapy which is a mainstream treatment ("Naturopathy," 2021).

It has to be noted that natural medicine is derived from age-old practices and studies, the philosophy of this field relies on the knowledge of old folk medicine and practices. It cannot be called evidence-based medicine (EBM) like that in the case of allopathy. There are still some practitioners who believe in EBM and try to work on the principles of evidence and proof.

TAKING CARE OF THE SICK

How a person is taken care of is what speeds or slows the recovery process. In recent times, what people generally do when they feel even a slight sickness is to pop a pill and then let the medicine take its due course in relieving them from the symptom.

Understandably, this is not a sound practice. Taking unprescribed medicine every single time you suffer from a slight headache is not the right approach toward your overall health and can actually cause internal damage in the long run. This should not just be the case with conventional medicines; while having herbal medicines, too, you must realize that consultation with a good practitioner is always the best to do.

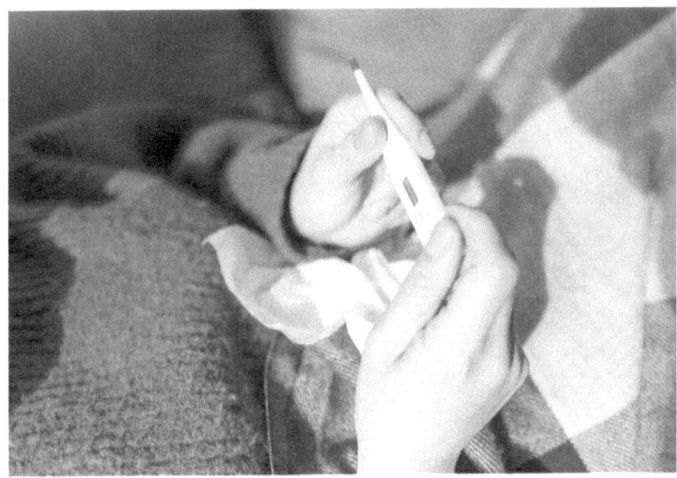

However, there are a few home remedies that you could try instead of consuming medicines of any form right away.

Home Remedies for Sore Throat and Cough

When you have that itch in your throat and a cough that seems to incessantly bother you, there are numerous home remedies that you can attempt before trying out other conventional medicines. As a professional medical provider, Sloun (2015) states:

I wish that being a doctor meant that my family and I would never get sick. Unfortunately, viruses, bacteria and other sources of illness do not discriminate based on profession. Here's what's in my toolkit to keep us going in sickness and in health. (para. 1)

Sloun (2015) discusses natural remedies that can be used for treating some health illnesses:

- Tea: Consuming hot tea can give you instant relief from an itchy and sore throat. There are ingredients called slippery elm and licorice that have throat-coating properties that have beneficial effects in reducing irritation of the throat.
- Honey: Said to have antibiotic and throat-coating properties that have been proven to cure cough and throat problems, you can take it with a spoon or mix it in warm water or tea. Be careful to not give honey to infants and toddlers as it might cause serious harm.
- Elderberry syrup: This is a remedy that has been used for centuries to cure colds and influenza.
- Echinacea: This can be used as a remedy to cure a cold by using drops and pills containing it.
- Pelargonium: This is a plant that is used to cure colds and coughs.

Home Remedies for Sleep

Sleep issues can create serious havoc in your daily life. Instead of trying strong medications that can be harsh for your system, you can try these two methods (Sloun, 2015):

- Tea: Try sipping some chamomile tea before your sleep time. It will relax your system and soothe your mind, which will, in turn, encourage a night of good sleep.
- Lavender: Lavender is known for its soothing properties. It can be used as an aromatherapy oil to calm your mind and relax your body. It has a relaxing effect that will induce you to sleep in no time.

Home Remedies for Digestion

One of the most common health issues that people face is concerning their digestion. Whether it is the food that is consumed or the quantity that is taken in, digestive problems can be painful and annoying. Here are a few remedies that you can try the next time you feel your stomach is a bit upset (Sloun, 2015):

- Ginger: This has been used by sailors for a very long time to cure nausea due to seasickness. It has medicinal properties and can be helpful in motion sickness and stomach problems. You can consume ginger by making small tablets of it at home or by drinking it in the form of tea.
- Probiotics: These are yeasts and bacteria that are termed "good bacteria." These are great for your digestive system and can help prevent stomach issues, especially diarrhea caused by the use of antibiotics or infections. These can be found in local stores in the form of miso paste, yogurt, kimchi, kombucha, and other fermented foods.

Home Remedies for Anxiety

Anxiety is an issue that countless people suffer from. Here are a few methods that you can use to lessen its effect:

- Do simple breathing exercises for a while every single day and while doing so, be grateful for everything good in your life.

- Slowly inhaling and exhaling breathing exercises can help calm you down instantly.
- Nourish your body with healthy food and juices.
- Keep your mind fresh by feeding in positive thoughts.

Home remedies can be highly beneficial in helping relieve some pain and health problems. Next time you feel uncomfortable with some sickness, you should head into your kitchen and grab some of those home remedy ingredients instead of popping those strong pills. Here are a few ingredients that have immense healing properties ("Home Remedies: What Works?" 2021):

- Peppermint: Mint has remarkable healing properties and has been used for generations to cure stomach-related issues. Irritable bowel syndrome that causes gas, diarrhea, bloating, cramps, and constipation can be relieved healthily by the use of some peppermint oil.
- Turmeric: Turmeric has been used as a medicine in many ways for numerous

years. It is used in cuts and wounds as an antibacterial measure. It is also said to help in fatty liver and arthritis conditions. It has been used to cure skin problems like rashes and ulcers.

- Garlic: It is widely believed that people who consume more garlic are less prone to certain types of cancer. Many use it to lower cholesterol and blood sugar as well.

Amazingly, you can see how many different natural items can prove to be beneficial for your entire health. The first step toward good health is acknowledging the fact that taking care of your mind and body is the key method. Negligence of health can lead to disastrous problems. However, with the correct use of herbal and natural medicines, you can prevent many issues concerning health.

Medicinal Plants for First Aid

Medicinal plants in the countryside, and even in some parts of the bigger cities, are not scarce. Nature has provided a plethora of plants and herbs that are highly effective at healing when used properly. According to clinical herbalist Steve Byers (as cited in Sarnacki, 2019), you do not need a ready-made band-aid to heal your wounds, you need to be connected to your land and use your resources effectively. Sarnacki (2015) talks about how these few medicinal plants that can be lifesaving when you are in the outdoors and have no access to any conventional medicine:

- Old Man's Beard: This plant is known as bearded lichen and is traditionally used for having antibacterial properties. It can be found throughout North America and its scientific name is *Usnea*. It is soaked in water and used on wounds, and it is also dried and powdered to be used externally.
- Cattails: This plant can help relieve burn wounds and is found widely in North America.
- Jewelweed: This plant can help in case of itching and pain caused by stinging nettle and poison ivy.
- Common Plantain: It can be mashed, made into a poultice, and used on wounds. It is found in North America and is known for its properties to soothe the skin.
- Calendula: Calendula is also found in

North America. It can be used as tea and can help in washing wounds. It is used extensively throughout the world to cure skin rashes, dry skin problems, bee stings, and inflammation.

- Common Yarrow: This plant is remarkable in stopping blood. It is one of the most kept in the first aid kit of wilderness explorers. It can be used to cure burns and wounds, and can at the same time, treat headaches and colds.
- Arnica: This plant is found in North America and is known to help in bruises and sprains.
- White Willow: The bark of this tree is said to have anti-inflammatory effects. It helps reduce headaches and other pain.
- Goldenseal: This plant is used to treat ear and skin infections.

As you can see, nature has provided remedies for every possible health issue, many of which are discovered and many of which are yet to be known. There is a magnanimous range of plants, and especially medicinal plants, that most of the time people hardly bother to understand or contemplate their value.

As a person who has seen a larger part of the world through the wilderness, one thing that has been a learning lesson is that nature can always be used in your favor in terms of medical emergencies. You will just have to be sure as to which plants to use precisely to help resolve a medical urgency. However, with the required knowledge, almost anyone can start on their journey to venture out in the wild without any fear or confusion.

4

UNDERSTANDING THE HUMAN ORGANISM

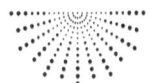

nderstanding the basics of survival and especially if you want to become a medical asset in the long run, help save lives. Additionally, at the same time to survive in the wilderness, you must understand how the human body works.

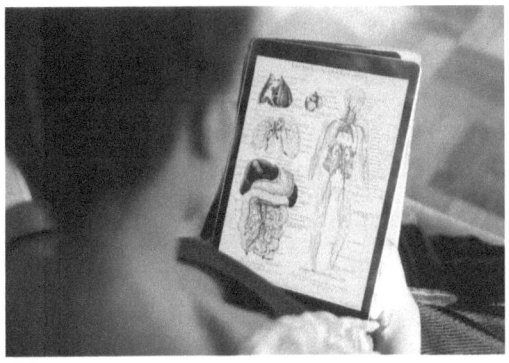

How many times do we even think about our body and wonder how it is designed and how it functions in the way it does? Hardly does anyone give a thought about these things. However, the main idea is that gaining vast knowledge about human anatomy will help you in many situations. With an adept knowledge of the human body, your problem-solving skills will be higher when it comes to anything related to humans and that is essential for survival.

OVERVIEW OF HUMAN ANATOMY

Human anatomy is a complex subject to understand fully, and many medical institutions require multiple semesters to complete this subject. Every bone, muscle, organ, blood vessel, and cell have their unique part to play in the design and function of the body. There are approximately 206 bones in the human skeleton, 600 muscles, 78 organs, and numerous cells and blood vessels ("Bones, Muscles, and Joints," 2012). The word anatomy means the study of the structure of living organisms and is a branch of medicine and biology. Therefore, studying and having clear knowledge of anatomy and an understanding of how all the major systems work is of prime importance for the study of medicine.

Skeleton

Skeleton is responsible for protecting all the vital organs and at the same time, giving a firm posture to the human body. The human body is moving all the time, whether walking, running, exercising, and even when resting, the human body is always functioning.

Fibrous connective tissues called ligaments are responsible for attaching the bones. Joints can be classified into two different types, movable and immovable based on their function. For example, movable joints can move and are flexible whereas immovable joints are not movable and are also called fixed joints.

Muscles

Muscles are tissues that assist the bones in locomotion. It is the tendons that connect the muscles to the bones. Movable bones function with the help of joints, but joints and bones cannot budge without the assistance of a muscle. Contracting and relaxing actions are used by muscles to propel the body forward.

Divisions of Human Anatomy

There are two important divisions in human anatomy:

- Macroscopic or gross anatomy: This division deals with structures that are large and that are visible to the naked eyes. This branch of study shows the location of all the human structures and also explains in detail how each structure is connected with the other.
- Microscopic anatomy: This division deals with the structures that are at the microscopic level, which means they are not visible to the naked eye. It is the second division of the study of human anatomy. It mainly studies tissues, veins, microscopic arteries, capillaries, and nerves, along with their position and role in the organ system.

Human anatomy is a vast subject to study. Therefore, a proper understanding of the different body parts can be studied in a systematic way to make it a bit easier.

Human Body Parts

The head, neck, and limbs are connected to the torso. Four limbs are perfectly postured to fit in the torso of the body. The shape of the body is given by the skeleton and is composed of bones and cartilage. All the organs of the body are placed inside the skeleton. Some of the relevant organs are the brain, heart, and lungs. The spinal cord is a very important component that connects the body with the brain.

Human Body Structure

The human body is composed of different cavities that are responsible for housing various organs. The three most distinct cavities are as follows:

- The cranial cavity: This cavity is responsible for the protection of the nervous system. It is a location in the skull where the brain and other important parts of the nervous system are firmly and safely placed. It acts as a shield to protect the brain from any external jerk or blow.

- The pleural cavity: This cavity is responsible for maintaining the optimal function of the lungs. It also acts like a protective wall that helps the lungs stay safe even when there is heavy breathing.
- The abdominal cavity: This is a cavity that is responsible for housing and giving external protection to the organs like the liver, spleen, and intestines.

These different cavities act as a support system for all the essential organs.

Circulatory System

The cardiovascular system of the human body is also referred to as the circulatory system. The heart and blood vessels including arteries, veins, and capillaries, are all an integral part of this system. There are two types of circulation systems:

- pulmonary circulation
- systemic circulation

The circulatory system is responsible for providing nutrients and oxygen to all the cells in the body. It also plays an integral part in removing waste and carbon dioxide. The heart is the organ that functions as a pumping machine to deliver oxygenated blood and deoxygenated blood to the required locations. Thus, it is also referred to as the transport system of the body.

Digestive System

Food is essential for the human body to function, and it is the digestive system that has the job of breaking down food and helps in supplying nutrients. These nutrients are further used by the body to repair its cells and for growth.

Descending in order, the most important parts of the digestive system are:

- mouth
- teeth
- tongue
- esophagus
- stomach
- liver
- pancreas

- gastrointestinal tract
- small and large intestines
- rectum

As simple as it may sound, the digestion process starts from the time you chew your food in your mouth. The saliva helps to soften the food which makes it easier to swallow. The chewed food then moves through the esophagus and enters the stomach. It is in the stomach that the most important part of the digestion takes place. Certain acids and enzymes are powerful enough to turn all the food into a paste.

After the process of the stomach, the food is moved into the small intestine. This is where food is digested even more because of a strong secretion that is released from the liver and pancreatic enzymes. It is at this stage that nutrients from the food get absorbed into the system. All the leftover material is moved to the large intestine where liquid is removed. Finally, all these materials are passed on through the rectum as waste in the form of stool.

Reproductive System

Commonly known as the genital system, the

reproductive system is a vital part of the human body. It is the most essential section that comprises all the external and internal organs that are responsible for reproductive function in humans. However, there are a few distinctions between the male and female reproductive systems. Understanding both reproductive systems will give you a transparent view on the distinctions and how each organ works toward the reproduction process in humans:

- Female Reproductive System: This is composed of ovaries and the uterine tubes. Ovaries are responsible for the production of female eggs called the ovum. It also produces a hormone called estrogen. Uterine tubes consist of fallopian tubes and oviducts. Also known as the womb, the uterus is a pear-shaped organ where the fetus grows. The cervix is between the uterus and the vagina. The vagina is where the male reproductive part, the penis, enters the female body during intercourse, delivering sperm that travels up through the cervix. This also acts as an exit for the fetus during the time of a normal delivery.
- Male Reproductive System: This consists

of testicles that store sperm that are essential for reproduction. These organs are oval and are placed in the scrotum. Vas deferens are muscular tubes located near the testis. This is one of the most important ducts belonging to the male reproductive system. Every time sperm is created, fluids produced by the seminal, Cowper's, and prostate gland merge. The Cowper gland then helps in increasing the volume of the semen that is required for lubrication during the process of coitus.

The reproductive system is an integral part of the human body system. It is because of this system that humans can generate offerings and carry on with the conventional process of life.

Nervous System

The nervous system is a complicated network of cells and nerves that are responsible for transporting signals from the brain and the spinal cord to all the different parts of the human body. The nervous system can be divided into two integral parts:

- Central Nervous System (CNS): All the voluntary and involuntary actions that a human body is capable of doing are guided and controlled by the CNS. Every part of the body is connected through axons. The CNS consists of the forebrain, midbrain, and hindbrain.
- The forebrain consists of the hypothalamus, thalamus, and cerebrum. The cerebrum is said to be the largest part of the brain. Understanding languages, thinking, perceiving, motor functions, emotional, and even sexual functions are controlled by this part of the brain.
- The midbrain is associated with the brain stem, and it is because of this part that visual and auditory functions can work smoothly.
- The hindbrain is that part of the brain that connects the spinal cord to neurons.
- Peripheral Nervous System (PNS): This system comprises all the nerves that branch out from the spinal cord and brain. It consists of two systems, namely the somatic and autonomic nervous systems.
- The main function of the somatic nervous

system is to pass all the sensory and motor impulses from the CNS and bring them back again. This system is linked with limbs, the skeletal system, and other sensory organs.

- The primary function of the autonomic nervous system is to relay impulses from the CNS to the muscles and other organs of the body. This system requires the support of the person. It is because of this system that the body can protect itself from any sudden blows, attacks, and also during conditions where the body temperature gets exceedingly high.

The nervous system is highly significant in the process of the normal functioning of the body. It is by which the mind and the body work in sync together.

The human body has a very unique way of functioning, especially with the presence of numerous cells and different organs; the entire process seems to be more complicated to understand. Through a proper study of the anatomy of the human body, and by understanding how major organs and muscles work, you can find it much easier to practice any medical treatments on anyone if need be during an emergency. It is necessary to understand how a particular system works because only with the optimal knowledge about the human body can you move ahead with your goal of becoming a medical asset in the future. Let us now dive into details about a few categories of illnesses and the first aid approaches to deal with them all.

RESPIRATORY ISSUES

Respiratory issues are often not taken seriously by many people. For example, they walk for a mile and start panting or they may take a hike up the mountains and find it difficult to breathe. In both cases, they will try and blame the exercise or the altitude for their breathing issues. Though they may be correct in their opinion, the fact is that breathing problems have to be taken seriously and taken care of in time before any complications crop up.

Breathing problems can be categorized into the following types:

- short of breath
- gasping for air because of inability to take deep breaths

- feelings of inadequate air supply

Breathing difficulty can be caused due to internal issues. Therefore, ensure you go through a thorough check-up if you notice any of the above symptoms regularly.

HEART ISSUES

Cardiac issues can be lethal if not taken care of at the right time. Some of the most common heart issues that you can encounter are a heart attack, sudden cardiac arrest, and an angina attack. Heart attacks can take place at any time, but there are a few symptoms that you have to be mindful of understanding.

One of the most prevalent symptoms of a cardiac arrest is that of chest pain. The pain generates in between your chest and then moves toward your neck, jaws, ears, arms, and wrists. The pain can be acute and initially, it will start with a mild ache. Sensations like heaviness, tightness, squeezing, constriction, and burning are some of the most common that you will feel. Most often, people confuse it with the sensation that is felt during heartburn or indigestion.

The following are some of the indicators of a cardiac arrest ("What to Do in an Emergency," 2020):

- chest pain
- pain in arms, jaw, neck, abdomen, and back.
- feeling sick
- sweaty
- looking pale
- restlessness and panicky
- breathlessness
- wheezing
- coughing
- rapid heartbeat, palpitation
- feeling dizzy

There are many cases where a woman or a diabetic may not feel any chest pain at all. However, if you spot any of the symptoms, then make sure you consult your doctor immediately.

Actions to Take During a Heart Attack

Call your local emergency number immediately! Make the patient sit and rest for some time until the ambulance arrives. Aspirin is said to be beneficial at such times but if you do not have it around, do not go searching for it as that time may be crucial not to be wasted. If you get an aspirin, chew a 300 mg aspirin immediately. Do not let the patient or even if it is you, stay alone until the ambulance arrives ("What to Do in an Emergency," 2020).

Once the paramedics arrive, give them all the medical details about the patient including allergies and medical history.

URINARY TRACT INFECTIONS

Urinary tract infection (UTI) is very common in people of all ages. This type of infection can occur in any part of your urinary system. The urethra, ureters, kidneys, and bladder can all be targets of this infection. Urine is said to contain no bacteria and is a byproduct of the kidneys. The process by which kidneys remove excess water from the waste material is what forms urine. Bacteria can enter the system from external sources and can cause inflammation and infection in the urinary tract.

Some of the most common symptoms of a UTI are:

- urinating frequently

- feel like urinating now and then
- pain during urinating
- lower back and side pain
- pain during intercourse
- fatigue
- pain in the penis
- fever
- vomiting
- confusion

It is believed that one in five women contracts a UTI every single year ("Urinary Tract Infections," 2010). UTIs are diagnosed by urinalysis and urine culture tests. Antibiotics are the most common way to treat UTIs. Some of the common antibiotics used are amoxicillin, doxycycline, quinolones, sulfonamides, nitrofurantoin, and many others. It is important to keep your body fluid up and not dehydrate yourself so, drink a lot of water.

GENITAL ISSUES

Infection of the reproductive organs can be termed genital issues. Such infections can affect all genders. However, let us take a look at what genital issues are for the male and female reproductive system distinctively.

Female Genital Infection

Female genital infections can be felt in the form of vaginal and yeast infections. If you have a vaginal yeast infection, you could try a home medication by using a non-prescription drug like tioconazole, clotrimazole, or miconazole. If your symptoms persist even after a few days, make sure to consult your doctor immediately.

Here are some of the ways to handle the situation:

- If you are pregnant, ensure that you consult your doctor immediately if you notice unusual vaginal symptoms.
- Avoid intercourse during the time of infection as that might cause you immense irritation and pain.
- Do not scratch the infected areas no matter how bad they itch.
- Apply cold compress to the affected area, cold baths can also help.
- Warm baths are said to help heal some

pain and itching.
- Wear cotton-made loose fitting clothes at all times.

Most vaginal infections clear up within a span of a few days. If you notice any of these symptoms, then visit your doctor soon and get a thorough check-up.

Male Genital Infection

Men are prone to genital infection as well. They are susceptible to yeast infection which can cause situations like balanitis. Swelling, pain, bruising, and inflammation are some of the common signs of male genital infection. There are quite a few home treatments that can be used to promote healing which can cure the condition in a matter of a few days. However, if the pain and swelling persist, it is always recommended to visit a doctor very soon.

If you would like to give it some time and try some home remedies, then here are a few methods:

- Rest is essential and while doing so, ensure to protect the sore area.
- Use ice packs to help reduce the swelling.

You can apply the pack for around 15 to 20 minutes many times a day.
- Wear loose, cotton underwear to help protect the bruised area.

By following these simple methods and at the same time, maintaining good hygiene, such infections can be put aside.

BLEEDING

You might get caught in an accident or cut by even a sharp tiny leaf. Whatever the reasons may be, bleeding is something that everyone should know how to handle. Here are a few steps by which you can control bleeding:

- If you encounter someone who is bleeding profusely, make sure that you remove their clothes and debris from the areas of the wound. If large objects have seeped into the body, ensure not to remove them as doing that can make the person bleed more.
- Wear your gloves before cleaning up the wound.

- Place a sterile bandage on the wound and firmly press it to stop the bleeding.
- Place the patient in a comfortable place and position.
- If the blood seeps through the gauze, then do not remove it. Instead, add more bandages on top of it.
- Use a tourniquet, if you know how to use it, as it is said to be effective in controlling heavy bleeding.

Even after you apply all the first aid procedures, if the patient does not stop bleeding, then you have to somehow take them to the nearest emergency facility or call the local emergency number.

You will experience a feeling of worth and contentment when you help save someone's life. Understanding the human body and how it works is fundamental knowledge that every person should have, but most importantly, someone who has prospects of getting into the healthcare business or making a career in the wild. The zeal that is required to learn human anatomy and work accordingly in emergencies can be very beneficial. Preparation is the key, and if you are prepared, you can win any battle in life.

5

HEADACHES, DENTAL CARE, AND MORE

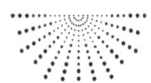

*H*eadaches and dental issues can be termed as minor in comparison to many of the dangerous diseases, but trust me on this, these two aches can make you suffer the most! You must have felt the pain of a headache if not a toothache. Both are equally difficult on the body and the pain is somewhat excruciating.

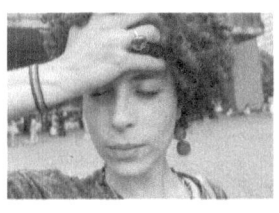

These types of aches happen anytime without any warning or previous symptoms and can cause havoc for quite some time. The fact is that there might be numerous underlying causes of such aches. Hence, understanding the root cause of the aches has to be done thoroughly. By doing so, you will be able to understand and also at the same time will be able to cure it accordingly.

Staying out in the sun for too long, having a heated discussion, tension, worries, and even loud noises can immediately give you severe headaches. Sometimes if you drink something cold or hot and also when the weather outside is very cold, you tend to get those bad toothaches. The cause may be many, but it is a worthwhile decision to dive into what and why these aches have been troubling you.

HEADACHES

According to the World Health Organization (2019), each person in the world suffers headaches every once in a while. The severity and duration vary, as well as the underlying cause.

Types of Headaches

Let us look at the different types of headaches that there are:

- tension
- migraine
- allergy and sinus

- hormone
- hypertension
- post-traumatic
- exertion
- caffeine
- cluster

In all the different causes of headaches, two of the most common forms of headaches are chronic headaches and episodic headaches. Chronic headaches can last for days and months; this type requires serious medical attention and pain management treatment. Episodic headaches on the other hand can last thirty minutes and up to eight hours. The pain in this case comes and goes quite often.

How to Cure Headaches

- Drink water: Staying hydrated can help you with the pangs of headaches. Sometimes due to dehydration, you can feel intense pain in your head. Drink enough water every day and keep your body nourished at all times.
- Limit alcohol: Alcohol can tweak the normal function of the brain for some

time, or rather while its intoxication remains. It is said that consuming alcohol can trigger migraine issues to a certain extent. Not just migraines: Alcohol can work like a diuretic, which can cause loss of fluid from the body that can eventually lead to dehydration, which again can worsen headaches.

- Use essential oils: The use of essential oils can be extremely therapeutic. Peppermint and lavender are two of the most used essential oils for headaches. Just take a few drops of the oils and rub them on your temples. It is one of the most natural and effective ways of lessening the effect of migraines.

- Apply a cold compress: If your head is burning with a headache, giving it a cold compress can help soothe the pain to a large extent. Place an ice gel or pace on the forehead and the neck regions; you will feel relieved in a matter of a few minutes.

- Drink coffee or tea: Some may find it bizarre, but it is a fact that drinking caffeinated tea can help soothe the pain of a headache. By consuming tea and coffee, the effectiveness of ibuprofen and acetaminophen increases. Ginger tea helps in soothing headaches as well.

- Try yoga: The healing properties of practicing yoga cannot be undermined. It is an effective way to release stress and can help in lessening the intensity of your headaches. According to a recent study, it has been found that practicing yoga for three months continuously resulted in a substantial decrease in the frequency of headaches (Kisan et al., 2014).
- Herbal Remedies: Certain herbal plants have the potential to soothe headaches. You can use feverfew and butterbur roots to help you cure the pain in your head (Stickler, 2020).

Many people suffer from headaches almost every moment of their lives. Headaches can cause not just severe pain, but because they can happen anytime and anywhere, they can also interfere with your plans. Imagine you are on a trip and have plans to do a lot during that period and migraine attacks frustrate you all of a sudden. Such situations are normal, and problems can happen almost any time in life.

However, by using effective home remedies for your headache problems, you can soothe your head and mind to a great extent. Ensure you carry a pain relief balm and a good painkiller that can effectively give you immediate relief in no time.

TOOTHACHES

The pain that you feel when chewing or drinking something cold or hot, is called toothache. Gum irritation and infections are the topmost cause of toothaches that people suffer from. More often, the deepest reasons for a toothache can be decaying or even chipping of the tooth due to cavities. In such cases, it is recommended that you visit your dentist as soon as possible.

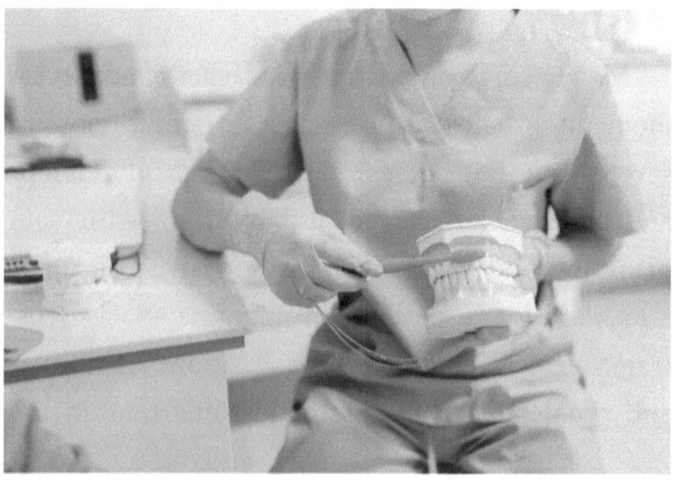

Dental care is important not just because teeth are situated at the face and can be visible; it is also important because stronger teeth can help you eat your food, which is essential to stay healthy in the long run. Additionally, neglectful teeth care can also eventually cause other health issues such as cardio-vascular disease, dementia, respiratory issues, infertility, and kidney disease, to name a few ("10 Health Issues Caused by Bad Oral Health," 2021).

Toothaches Can Be Highly Painful

The nerves that are situated inside the pulp of your teeth are very sensitive. When these pulps get infected by bacteria, that can cause immense pain. Sometimes they are so sensitive that even a sip of cold coffee can generate pain that could last for days.

Causes of Toothaches

Toothaches can be caused due to several reasons. Some of these causes are as follows:

- Gum infection: Infection in the gum can cause swelling which can lead to severe pain for a very long time.

- Tooth decay: Decaying of the tooth is one of the most common reasons for toothaches. Teeth become vulnerable when they are covered with cavities and decay, causing pain now and then.
- Abscessed tooth: Bacterial infection can occur in the insides of the tooth which can result in pain and swelling of the gums.
- Tooth fracture: When the tip of the tooth chips off or gets half-broken, then that can create severe problems. The chipped tooth can sometimes hurt and cut the inner linings of the cheeks causing infection, which again can result in acute pain.
- Tooth repair: There are times when you get your tooth fixed but then later damage can occur after some time. Visit your dentist regularly and get your dental work checked.
- Rigorous chewing: Chewing on hard items can weaken the teeth from the roots. The impact of chewing continuously can be severe in terms of the health of the teeth. Something as normal as chewing a piece of gum for a long period can result in massive jaw and tooth pain.

- Eruption: Recent tooth surgery or any tooth procedure can result in swelling and pain for days. Most often dentists even recommend patients to go on a liquid diet for a few days to help heal the scars faster.

People of all ages are susceptible to problems related to teeth. Toothaches are common, and different techniques are used to heal the problem and soothe the pain for many years. Let's discuss a few methods by which you can overcome your toothaches at home.

Natural Ways to Heal Toothaches

There are many reasons that cause toothaches, but instead of jumping right in with strong medicines as a relief, you can try some of these effective home remedies (Ponsford, 2017):

- Cold compress: Most toothache problems are caused due to injured, infected gums or tooth decay. Every time you get a pain in your tooth, place an ice pack or a cold compress on top of the cheeks below the painful tooth. By applying a cold compress, you can slow down the process of blood circulation in the painful area. Apply it a couple of times and you will be able to feel the difference.

- Garlic: A compound called allicin is present in garlic which gives it medicinal value. This compound has strong antibacterial properties and can have healing effects. You can crush the garlic with a pinch of salt and apply it directly to the affected tooth.

- Saltwater mouthwash: This is an age-old practice that most people have been following for a very long time. Take some warm water and add some salt to it, stir it well and sip and keep it in your mouth for some time. By rinsing with warm salt water, debris attached to the cavities will also get washed off and will at the same time reduce swelling of the gums. You can repeat it as many times as you need to.

- Peppermint tea: Peppermint tea has a numbing effect and when applied to the tooth, it can diffuse the pain in no time. You can use peppermint oil or prepare a solution mixed with a teaspoon of peppermint boiled in water. You can use this water to rinse your mouth occasionally.

- Clove oil: Clove oil has a numbing effect. It is readily available in the market. You can apply a drop of it on the affected tooth, but make sure to apply it with cotton and in small quantities. This is because clove oil can have a hot effect on the skin if used more.

- Aloe vera: Aloe vera gel is used mainly in conditions of cuts and burns. In recent times, people have started using it for toothaches. This is because it has antibacterial properties and can destroy germs that cause tooth decay.

- Hydrogen peroxide rinse: First of all, this solution has to be used with extra caution as it should never be swallowed. However, it has antibacterial properties because rinsing your mouth with it can help cure gum infections.

- Thyme: Thymol is a component of the essential oil that has vital antiseptic and antibiotic properties. These properties make it known for medicinal purposes.

Just a drop of thyme oil in water and rinsing your mouth with it can do the trick.

Visit a Dentist

Herbal medicines and home remedies can help you get some relief from your toothache problems. Avoid eating food that has hard textures. Sugary food items can also aggravate pain. If pain and swelling last for more than a few days, then consult with your dentist immediately for treatment and regular checkups.

INSOMNIA

Insomnia is a sleep disorder that keeps you awake and even if you do manage to fall asleep, then it is only for a fleeting moment. Just the way the human body needs proper nourishment and exercise, sleep is equally important, too. Insomnia is a condition that not only disrupts your lifestyle and regular work but can also drain all your energy and make you perpetually exhausted.

The majority of adults require a minimum of seven to eight hours of sleep. Sleep issues are a common problem. Many may experience insomnia for a short-term that may last for a few days whereas some may experience insomnia that lasts for months on end. In any of the cases, insomnia can be caused due to many reasons, like traumatic experiences or some underlying health conditions.

Symptoms and Causes of Insomnia

Insomnia may result because of many problems. Some of the prominent signs and underlying reasons of insomnia are as follows ("Insomnia," 2016):

- difficulty in falling asleep
- no sound sleep
- waking up in between sleep
- waking up after a few hours
- exhausted even after sleeping
- work schedule
- excessive travel
- eating late at night
- depression, anxiety, and irritable mood swings
- feeling of sleepiness during the day
- lack of attention
- lack of focus

- caffeine and nicotine consumption
- alcohol consumption
- dull memory
- loop of worries about not having sleep

These points mentioned are all self-explanatory. If you face any of these issues, you must pay attention to where you are going wrong in your habits. Try to instill habits that will help you focus on a healthy lifestyle that can boost your sleeping habits.

There are a few other causes that could be related to the condition of insomnia ("Insomnia," 2016):

- Mental Health Disorders: Traumatic events in life can cause major sleep disorders. Feelings of anxiousness can cause severe stress and exhaustion that can adversely affect your sleeping habits.
- Medications: Some medications can cause problems in sleeping habits. Some medicines may have sedatives that could make you fall asleep, whereas some medicines contain stimulants and caffeine that could again disrupt sleep.
- Medical Conditions: Many chronic diseases have been linked with insomnia

like diabetes, cancer, asthma, heart disease, overactive thyroid, Alzheimer's, and Parkinson's disease.

- Sleep-Related Disorders: Restless leg system syndrome and sleep apnea can cause major sleep disturbances.

Visit a Doctor

You can be living with insomnia for months and may be confusing it with mere feelings of anxiety or a condition of exhaustion. If you notice that your lack of proper sleep is hampering your regular life and work and is getting way beyond any control, then you must realize that it is time for you to consult with a doctor. You must understand the underlying cause of your lack of sleep. If by any chance your doctor concludes that you are suffering from a sleep disorder problem, then they will send you to a sleep center for further tests. Getting a thorough screening of your health done is beneficial. Staying focused and prepared for any situation is the best way to tackle things.

Those at Risk of Insomnia

According to the Mayo Clinic (2016), there are categories of people who are at a higher risk for insomnia:

- Over the age of 60: If you are above the age of 60, then chances are that you may be a victim of insomnia. This is because with age, sleep patterns and health conditions change and fluctuate which results in disturbance in sleep habits.
- Women: If you're a woman, then the hormonal changes that happen during the menstrual cycle and mainly during menopause, can cause severe sleep disorders. Insomnia is more common in pregnant women. The hot flashes and night sweats tend to cause disturbances in sleep.
- Mental disorder: Mental issues that result in anxiety, panic attacks, exhaustion, and frustration can all lead to a condition of loss of sleep.
- Stressed: Stress is a major factor that affects your health and most importantly, your sleep.
- Erratic schedule: Working in irregular

shifts and having a messy routine can add
to a habit of sleeping late that could
eventually make its way toward insomnia.

Insomnia can cause tons of issues in your personal as well as your professional life. From not paying attention at work to becoming irritable and spoiling the mood of everyone around you, detrimental behavior can add up to some of the problems. With lack of sleep, you can even risk your health from acute diseases, mainly cardiovascular diseases, in the future.

Remedies That Help Insomnia

Insomnia can be controlled by instilling good sleeping habits. Here are a few ways in which you can keep your insomnia at bay ("Insomnia," 2016):

- Set a bedtime and make sure that you
  follow your routine of sleeping and
  waking up at the right time. Continue this
  process for a few weeks, and you will
  notice a vast difference in your sleep
  timings.
- Having an active day can help you rest

well at night. Do not be a couch potato, even if it is for half an hour, make sure that you take a walk around the house or in your office area. Physical activity done during the day can help your muscles rest well at night.

- Refrain from taking naps during the day. By taking short naps in the day, you can disrupt your sleep pattern which can make you fall asleep very late at night.
- Do not eat large meals and drinks before bedtime.
- Take a warm bath before sleep and set your bed in a very comfortable way that could induce you to sleep.

Insomnia is not simply about losing your sleep, it adds to the regular functions of your life. It is not at all healthy to lose sleep, no matter what the reasons may be. Your health is in your hands, so make an effort to work your way through this problem and come out of it successfully by being insomnia-free.

CHRONIC FATIGUE

Chronic fatigue syndrome is a condition in which you experience extreme fatigue for a very long duration. Sometimes, this syndrome can last for more than six months at a time. The problem with this condition is that it cannot be cured with rest and is also tricky to diagnose.

Symptoms of Chronic Fatigue

Some of the most common signs and symptoms of chronic fatigue disorder are as follows:

- dim memory and concentration level
- sleep that does not make you feel refreshed
- dizziness when standing from a sitting posture and sitting from a lying posture

There are other symptoms that are said to be related to this condition like fatigue, sore throat, headaches, unexplained pain in the body, and enlarged lymph nodes in the armpits and neck regions.

Causes of Chronic Fatigue

Although, it is difficult to point to a particular reason for this bizarre medical condition like the chronic fatigue syndrome, here are a few potential causes that can lead to this condition ("Chronic Fatigue Syndrome," 2020):

- Viral infections: Many people get chronic fatigue syndrome after having a viral infection. Some researchers believe that a few types of viruses may be the cause of such an issue. Epstein-Barr virus and human herpes virus 6 are suspected to be the viruses involved.
- Hormonal imbalance: Hormonal imbalance has been noticed in people who have chronic fatigue syndrome. Correlations between the two have not been found, just speculation that these two issues could be related and could be causing the problem.
- Immunity problems: There is speculation whether chronic fatigue syndrome can be caused due to weak immunity. The people

who suffer from this syndrome seem to have an impaired immune system.

- Emotional or physical trauma: A sudden stress or trauma could be some of the reasons for getting chronic fatigue syndrome. Many people have reported that they got this syndrome after they encountered surgery, injury, or any form of emotional trauma.

Visit a Doctor

Fatigue in general is not taken as a serious concern. A few days of rest and usually, you are good to go. However, in the case of chronic fatigue syndrome, feeling tired can last for days and months. Therefore, if you notice any of the mentioned symptoms along with a long period of unexplained fatigue, then ensure to consult with your doctor immediately.

6

BONES AND JOINTS

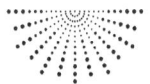

*B*ones and joints have a crucial part to play in the functioning of the human body. Bones are responsible for giving strong support to the entire body. People are shaped by their bones. They support the body and safeguard vital organs such as the heart and liver.

Bones contain marrow, which produces new blood cells, and stores the minerals calcium and phosphorus. Joints, on the other hand, are the parts of the 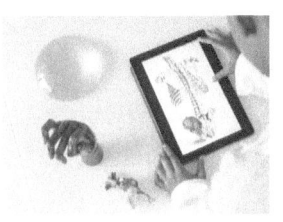 body where bones connect. They are responsible for attaching two or more bones together so that there is a smooth function of movement.

BONE STRUCTURE

Vertebrates are the only living creatures to have bones. Due to these bones, there is some rigidity in the body. Bones play a role in storing micronutrients and also bone marrow, both essential for life.

Bone is also called an osseous tissue which is a calcified connective tissue that constitutes the endoskeleton of the human body. A matrix of ground material and collagen fibers contains osteocytes. These cells are the most prevalent type of cell in adult bone, and they are in charge of bone development and density. Calcium and phosphate are abundantly stored in the bone matrix, which further strengthens and densifies the structure. Bones are differentiated based on their shapes and placement.

Long Bones

As the name itself implies, long bones are long, and they have two ends and a shaft. Bone marrow is contained in a marrow cavity in the diaphysis or middle shaft. The epiphyses are the rounded ends of the bones that are covered in articular cartilage and packed with red bone marrow that produces blood cells. The femur, tibia, radius, and ulna are all examples of long bones that make the majority of the limb structure.

Short Bones

Short bones are also known by the name of cuboidal bones. These bones are the same length and width, which gives them a cubical shape. The ankles and wrists consist of short bones.

Flat Bones

Flat bones are slender and relatively broad bones that are present where considerable organ protection or vast muscle attachment surfaces are required. The sternum is also known as the breastbone. The scapula or shoulder blades, ribs, and the roof of the skull are all examples of flat bones.

Irregular Bones

Bones that have irregular shapes and complex nature are called irregular bones. The surfaces of these bones are short, notched, flat, or ridged. The hip bones, vertebrae, and various skull bones are examples of irregular bones.

Sesamoid Bones

Sesamoid bones are tiny in size and resemble sesame seeds in shape. The patellae are also sesamoid bones. This type of bone grows inside tendons and can be found in feet, knees, and hand joints.

Sutural Bones

Irregularly shaped bones that are small and flat in size and shape are known as sutural bones. This bone can be detected between the flat skull bones. They all vary in shape, location, and size.

JOINT INTEGRATION

The point at which two or more bones connect is called a joint. A variety of fibrous connective tissue can be found in joints. Ligaments are the connective tissues that hold the bones together. The muscles of the bones are connected by tendons. It is the cartilage that protects the end of bones by cushioning them. There are two types of joints, and they are immovable and slightly movable joints. Let's understand how they function.

Immovable and Slightly Movable Joints

In this type of joint structure, there is no presence of the joint cavity. It is the collagen and the fibrous tissues that are responsible for connecting the bones. Interestingly, the bones of the skull of an infant are flexible in the beginning, but with time, the bones join together and calcify into becoming a bone. It is the fibrous tissues that are responsible for joining the teeth in the gums. The slightly movable joints refer to the cartilaginous joints in which the bones are stuck together by cartilage as there is no joint cavity.

Synovial Joints

Synovial joints are movable joints and are very common throughout the body. Different types of synovial joints can move in different ways. Joint capsules, or fibrous tissue, surround these joints. Synovial fluid is secreted from this capsule because of the way the spaces and tissues get lubricated inside the capsule.

Ball and Socket Joints

This is a type of joint that can move and rotate in many different ways. Ball and socket joints are found in the hip and shoulder of the body.

Condyloid Joints

Condyloid joints are found in the fingers and jaw. These joints are versatile and are movable, but they cannot rotate.

Gliding Joints

These are the joints that can glide around in the body, especially in the spine, wrists, and ankles.

Hinge Joints

The parts of the human body that bends, like the knees and elbows, are composed of this type of joint.

Pivot Joints

Your neck and elbow both have pivot joints, which allow bones to pivot or twist around other bones.

Saddle Joint

The best example of this type of joint is the thumb. It can move from side to side but cannot rotate.

Range of Motion

The bones and joints in the human body are connected in such a way that some can move fully whereas some can move only partially. The degree to which a joint can move is called the range of motion. For example, the degree to which your arms connected by your elbow can move is called the range of motion.

Two different categories fall under the range of motion:

- Extension: The bones connected with the joints are placed apart and also straightened from a bent angle. Due to this, the space and angle between the joint and the bones in the limbs are increased.
- Flexion: The bones are pulled together that form the joint. In this condition, the

angle and space between the joint and the bones of a limb are reduced.

CONDITIONS AFFECTING BONES AND JOINTS

There are several conditions that bones, and joints are susceptible to in terms of health-related issues.

Here are a few situations, or rather ailments, that are common:

Osteoarthritis

Arthritis is a condition that is associated with synovial joints. It is an inflammatory condition in which there is damage done to the cartilage over the years. Due to this, the cartilage thins down in the process and causes extreme pain between the bones.

Rheumatoid Arthritis

This is a condition that is associated with the immune system and its failure to save the tissues of the joints. In this autoimmune disease, the damage is done to the tissues which results in pain in the joints.

Gout

This condition is caused when the synovial joint is filled with uric acid crystals. The synovial membrane gets inflamed with use, which in turn, results in synovitis.

Fractures

Fractures are a condition when your bones get cracked or broken into a few pieces. This can be caused due to many reasons including, accident, fall, or any form of physical trauma. Although fractures are not usually a life-threatening problem, they do require an elaborate process of taking care of them. Fractures can be diagnosed with the help of an x-ray, but there are a few symptoms that could suggest a broken bone:

- excruciating pain in the injured area
- numbness in the same area
- visible swelling in the surrounding areas
- bluish color bruise
- bone protruding is seen through the skin
- heavy bleeding through the cut wound

There are different types of fractures:

- Stable: When the bone breaks but stays in its position.
- Transverse: When the fracture happens at a 90-degree angle of the bone.
- Comminuted: Most common after a trauma-like accident in which the bone gets shattered into many pieces.
- Oblique: When long bones like the femur break at an angle such that a deformity can be seen below the skin.
- Compound: Requires immediate surgery as the bone breaks and pierces through.
- Hairline: Stress fracture that happens mostly in the hands and feet due to rigorous movements like running or jogging.
- Greenstick: Only a portion of the brain breaks and also bends at the end.
- Spiral: When a bone breaks due to twisting of the limb.
- Pathological: When a patient has been ill and the bones get weakened as a result.

Fractures can happen anywhere at any time,

more so, if you are out in the wild. In case you find anyone who might have a fracture, you should take the following steps immediately until the emergency team arrives:

- Stop bleeding if there is a cut or a wound.
- Apply cold in the affected area.
- Immobilize the injured person and do not allow sudden movements.
- Prepare a sling that could hold the fractured part steady and safe.
- Use the nearest available bandages and a frame of sticks to keep the hurt part upright and in place without pulling or pushing hard.
- Call the doctor immediately

Sudden accidents are bound to happen, especially when you are in the wild. If you ever face a situation where someone in your group falls and the symptoms show that they must be suffering from a fracture, then even without any medical help around, you can create a cast or a splint for the patient to keep their injury safe in a correct position. Here are a few tips on how you can go about it:

- If the arms are hurt, take a firm cloth and use it carefully to wrap it around the elbow comfortably and take the cloth upward and slowly tie it around the neck. This will immediately help immobilize the injured hand.

- For a lower leg splint, you will need padded material, preferably a foam pad that you can cut from a sleeping pad and around three cravats or anything wide enough to wrap around the splint. You can use rope to tie it around. This will give support to the legs and can help them stay in position until the medical team arrives for proper medical tests.

- Birch bark is widely used to handle a broken bone situation in the wild. The technique is simple: peel off the skin of a tree and wrap it around the affected hand or leg like you would do while making a canoe. It has natural curls which makes it easy to wrap around. You can then use any bandage at your disposal to give it support.

- Sticks and even tent poles can be used to make a temporary splint.

- If you have notebooks that have hardcovers or sleeping mats, you could use those as a material to make a splint.
- Mud casts can also be used to assist and give support to broken bones. Check a riverbank or get some wet clay and wrap it around with the help of rolled gauze in the affected area. Wrap it around the affected limbs. Slowly wrap another layer of cloth or gauze to give it support. Do not make it very heavy, just the right weight to support the bone will be enough. This will act as a plaster to keep the injured bone safe.

When taken to the emergency center, numerous tests can give a clear picture of the bone damage. From x-rays to scanning, everything will be available. Bone scanning is also done to examine the health of the bone. It is usually done to check diseases of the bone including arthritis, bone cancers, avascular necrosis, fibrous dysplasia, infection, Paget's disease, and even fractures.

Sprains

When joints like the ligaments and wrists get twisted and hurt then that is called a sprain. Your ankle can get hurt when you walk or jog and accidentally twist your foot and stretch it so hard that the ligaments which support the ankles get hurt.

Sprains are considered to be minor, but they can be divided into three categories based on the level of the damage:

- Grade 1: When the ligaments are stretched but not torn. Such sprains will be healed within a day or two. These sprains are the most common of all the sprains.
- Grade 2: When the ligament is torn partially, and the doctor can feel it when you move your ankle. Such sprains take a time of six to eight weeks to heal.
- Grade 3: When the ligament is completely torn. Such sprains take a longer time to heal, like three to six months.

Symptoms of Sprained Ankle

Here are a few symptoms to detect if you have a sprained ankle:

- bruising
- pain
- swelling
- tenderness
- instability
- restricted motion
- popping sensation

Grade 1 sprains can be treated at home. Here are a few tips on how to handle an ankle ("Home Remedies for a Sprained Ankle," 2019):

- Apply ice on the affected area.
- Apply a crepe bandage loosely and keep it on until the swelling decreases.
- Turmeric has inflammatory properties. It can be mixed with lime juice, and a few drops of water can be made into a paste to apply to the sprained area. You can apply a bandage over it.
- Garlic can also be used to treat the symptoms of a sprain. One tablespoon of crushed garlic along with some coconut oil can be applied to the affected area to reduce inflammation and pain.
- Soak the sprained ankle in warm water

mixed with Epsom salt. This can have a healing effect.

- Arnica has healing properties beneficial for joints and muscles. Dilute arnica oil and gently apply it to the sprained area.
- Castor oil has pain-relieving properties and can be applied gently on the sprained portion.
- Cabbage compresses are used widely to help reduce swelling caused by a sprain.

Treating sprains can be easy and is possible without the help of a medical practitioner. It is only if the symptoms are unbearably painful that you should immediately call a doctor.

Torn Ligament

A band of fibrous tissue called ligament connects bone to bone and cartilages as well. Ligaments are not delicate but can be torn or stretched due to the sudden impact of certain joints and ankles. Sudden fall or sometimes even a high-intensity workout can lead to a ligament tear in the knees, ankles, wrists, neck, thumbs, and back.

Here are a few symptoms which indicate a case of ligament tear:

- excess pain
- tender to touch
- swelling
- bruising
- sound of pop during the time of the ligament injury

The torn ligament can be treated with ample rest, cold compress, and wrapping of crepe bandage over the affected area. Keep the ankle or the part of the body that is injured in an elevated position to control the blood circulation in that area. This will substantially reduce the swelling caused by the injury. However, if the pain persists and the swelling does not reduce after a day or two, call a doctor.

Helpful Tips

Situations can change in a minute when you are out in the wild. If you face any of the problems that we've discussed so far, it becomes imperative on your part to understand the different techniques and remedies that you could use to heal and provide the required first aid to someone who needs it the most.

Your knowledge about the human body and different illnesses can help you survive even the toughest of circumstances in the wild. From allergies to snake bites, from giving CPR to healing a wound, from making splints for an injured bone to treating various infections, you will require every bit of knowledge of medicine while you are out in the wild alone with no medical assistance nearby. The confidence that you gain through such knowledge will help you enjoy outdoor life. There will be no holding you back due to the fear of health issues. You will be prepared and will be able to handle even the most difficult situation with utmost care and calm.

7

CARING FOR OPEN WOUNDS

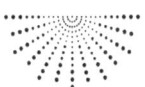

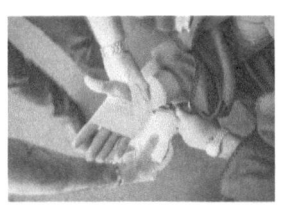pen wounds are always cause for concern whether you are facing them in the city or outdoors. There will be times when no matter how cautious you are while hiking or even doing a simple errand at home, you might get a cut which can result in an open wound.

Take for instance, when you're fixing your window-pane and a piece of wood breaks and slashes your arm with its sharp edge. It might happen so quickly that you may not see it coming at all. No doubt, due to the sharp edge, you will get a cut. Cuts, if left open, can cause severe hazards: you can bleed profusely, and at the same time, can get severe infections.

Similarly, in a rather difficult situation in the wilderness while hiking, if you get a severe cut, leaving it open can cause acute health hazards. It is profoundly important to deal with open wounds because these kinds of wounds are common. By gaining knowledge about how to prepare for a situation with open wounds, you can help prevent dangerous infections.

WHAT IS AN OPEN WOUND?

An open wound, as the name suggests, refers to an accident that has caused the internal and external body tissues to break. This type of wound is generally located near the skin area. From childhood to becoming an adult, almost everyone is bound to experience this type of wound sometime in their lives.

Most open wounds are treatable at home, but again, the depth and the size of the cut matter. Many times, when the cut is too deep, stitches will be required which can be provided by an experienced professional only. In such a case, it is best to visit the doctor as soon as possible. The treatment of open wounds depends on the type of the wound.

TYPES OF OPEN WOUNDS

Abrasion

When your body rubs against a coarse surface and gets scraped then that is called abrasion. You must have noticed when you fall or even during bike accidents, people get abrasions on their arms, hands, knees, limbs, and faces. Abrasions affect the outer layer of skin, therefore, there is no case of intense bleeding. Most of the time, such abrasions are cleaned with an antiseptic wash and then an ointment is applied. It needs to be lightly bandaged to avoid any external infection. In no time, such abrasions dry off and heal completely.

Puncture

When you get hit by a pointy object, it causes a puncture through the skin. When a person gets hit by a bullet, that also forms a puncture. The wound that is formed by a puncture can be very deep, harming internal organs. However, not much bleeding happens with minor punctures.

For wounds like this, you need to visit a medical practitioner and get tests done to see if there is any internal bleeding.

Laceration

Open wounds are caused by sharp objects like knives, machinery, and tools with sharp edges. This kind of cut can cause rapid and heavy bleeding. Therefore, the primary step to help is to make an effort to stop the bleeding immediately.

Avulsion

These are wounds caused due to violent accidents and explosions. Tearing of the skin and tissue makes this wound a painful one. The bleeding through such a wound can be very heavy, and you must immediately try and stop the bleeding of the person suffering from it.

TREATMENT OF OPEN WOUNDS

There is a wide range of treatments available for open wounds. The treatments depend on the type and depth of the wound. Some minor open wounds can be easily treated at home or anywhere outside.

However, wounds that are severe and which have a chance of getting a bad infection, must be treated immediately.

Home Remedies to Treat Open Wounds

Wounds have to be immediately washed off with a disinfectant liquid or any soap available. This will help clean the wound and prevent infections from spreading further. After you clean the wound from all the dirt and debris, make sure you place direct pressure on the opening to stop any bleeding.

Use an antibacterial or antibiotic ointment or gel and apply it gently over the injury. Place a light bandage over the top to keep it clean. Very small wounds do not require any bandaging.

There will be pain and some swelling; if they are mild, then you just need some good rest. For the pain, you can take a mild painkiller. Ensure that you avoid medicines like aspirin, as that can encourage more bleeding.

For the selling, you can use a cold compress of ice. If you are out in the woods, you will have to follow the same procedures, but one thing you could add is to apply a light layer of sunscreen on the area of injury to protect it from the harsh heat until it heals completely.

Know When to Call For Help

Minor wounds can be controlled and taken care of; what matters is when to realize that the wound is major. This is not a problem if you are near the reach of a health facility in the city but can be a huge problem if you are out in the wilderness.

Cuts and abrasions are common when you are on an expedition in the outdoors, but for wounds that are deep and acute, it is best to evacuate your position and head toward the nearest health center.

Here are a few reasons that should make you realize that it is time for evacuation from the outdoors:

- If the wound is big and needs sutures or stitches.

- If the wound contains debris that has seeped in it during the accident.
- If the wound has been caused by an animal attack. Animal paws and teeth can cause fatal infections.
- If there are symptoms like chills, fever, excessive swelling, and red bruises.
- If the wound is wide enough to expose the bones, especially the joints.
- If the cut is very deep and is on the face.
- If the wound has coverage of dead tissues around.
- If the bleeding does not stop even after trying all the first aid methods.
- If the wound is preventing any mobility.

If you are in the wild, one of the disadvantages that you face is the lack of proper cellular coverage. In times like this, it will be impossible for you to call anyone for help. One of the cautionary measures that you can take before setting on a trip in the wild is carrying two or three simple phones that have different network providers. Switch them off while you do not need them, but you can check if any of the networks can get a call through when the situation arises.

Stab Wound

Globally, the crime rate seems to be increasing by the day. There are numerous miscreants out there, of whom you can never be aware. Due to such reasons, sometimes traveling alone, and especially taking long expeditions by yourself, can be a bit risky. This thought, though, should not stop you from taking the trip that you've always wanted to or your desire to seek the wilderness. The point is that you must always be prepared to be safe and also should be aware of some of the most essential self-defense techniques

When you venture out in the wild, you must have a strong heart to face challenges and deal with the problems if there are any. For instance, you are on your way to mountainous terrain, and your car is approached by a person who has been stabbed and thrown on the road. Of course, your first step must be to immediately call the cops and ambulance. But while you wait for the help to arrive, you can do your bit to help the person survive.

It is evident that since you are on your journey to the outdoors, you will have your first aid kit with you. Here are a few ways to help a stabbed person:

- When you encounter a stabbed person, your primary concern will be to stop the bleeding. Never forget to wear your gloves before touching anything that has an opening or blood in it. Do not wash the injury because it is a major one, it will be given a thorough cleaning at the hospital.
- Make the person lie or sit in a comfortable position to avoid dizziness or fainting.
- Check if there is anything external stuck in the injury. If you find something in, do not attempt to remove it.
- Try to elevate the part that is injured above the heart to slow down the bleeding to some extent.
- Most important of all, apply direct pressure on the wound to stop heavy bleeding.
- Talk gently to the patient and make an effort to maintain the patient's full consciousness.

By taking care of the stabbed patient until the medical rescue team reaches the scene, can help them survive.

How to Close Wounds

Major wounds must always be treated at a hospital. However, if you do not find a way to reach any medical help soon, then closing a wound should be one of the last options.

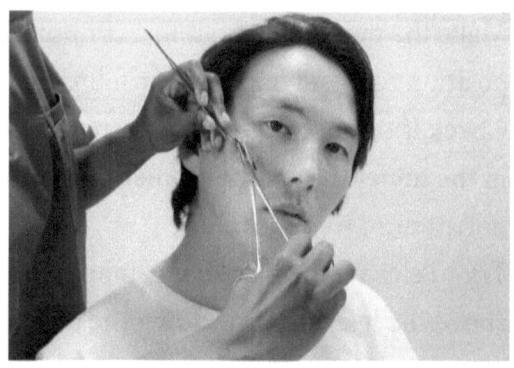

There are many different ways in which wounds can be closed and some of them are listed below

Staples

Surgical staples are considered to be a reasonable method to help close an open wound. This method can be used when there is no time to take the patient to a proper medical center on time. You can use staples quite quickly and this can be highly helpful in controlling bleeding. In cases of multiple wounds, this technique can be fast and efficient. Using surgical staples needs minimal training and can be highly cost-effective as well. If done correctly and hygienically, the healing time of this method is the same as sutures. Always ensure that the staple that you use is thoroughly sanitized to prevent any form of infection in the process.

Sutures

Sutures are a common and very old conventional method to seal a wound. Sutures are of two different types, absorbable and non-absorbable. Absorbable sutures are strong enough that the chemicals of the body will not be able to dissolve them. These sutures are mostly used in external wounds and cuts. However, for surgeries that require double layer closing, like in the case of uterus surgery, then absorbable sutures will work the best as there will be no requirement to open the sutures again. The choice of sutures that should be used completely depends on the nature of the wound.

In the case of long wounds, a running suture is said to be the most beneficial. For a deep wound, a mattress stitch can also be used as it is said to give stronger support to the wound.

Adhesives

Skin adhesive is the easiest and painless option that can be used to close an open wound. You can firmly but with a gentle hand, carefully place the adhesive on the cut and bring the skin together slowly and stick it with adhesive. Using adhesive narrows down your chance of getting an infection way more than sutures. The use of adhesives is the best option for a person who is out in the wild. However, here are a few things that you need to be cautious about while dealing with open wounds:

- Clean the area thoroughly before applying any form of suture or adhesive.
- Place the edges of the skin gently with each other and then apply the adhesive over it.
- Refrain from pulling the skin very hard to bring them closer. This can cause the wound to tear more.
- Finally, when the position is set correctly,

use a skin adhesive or glue to seal the
wound.

Be aware of the hygiene process and never touch a wound with anything dirty. Always carry an antiseptic wash and a cream with you. They are handy and can be used in many ways.

Healing Process

After the treatment of open wounds, the healing process can take a while and may be different for every individual. Many factors can slow down the process of healing. Ensure that you monitor the wound and give the appropriate dressing on time.

Factors like oxygen not reaching the wound through proper blood circulation can be one of the reasons why a wound may heal slowly. Such wounds can take double the time compared to a wound that receives adequate oxygen and nutrient supply through the blood. High blood sugar levels, blood pressure, and even obesity can slow down the process of healing.

Wound dressing is the key to clearing out a wound. Ensure you do it regularly by maintaining all the hygiene protocols; in just a matter of days, the wound will start drying up and eventually heal completely. Observe your patient for some time, and if the wound has developed an infection and is not healing fast enough, then make sure that you consult the doctor immediately.

8

TENDING TO THE PATIENT

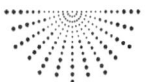

hen a patient goes through any trauma or sickness, there is a high probability that they will not behave the same as they would in normal circumstances. People are different, and it is their personal, mental, and physical capacity that can help them deal with a situation. As a medical asset, it is a requirement that you should know all the basics of medicine and treatment. However, the most challenging part of your job will be to deal with a panicky patient in a time of crisis.

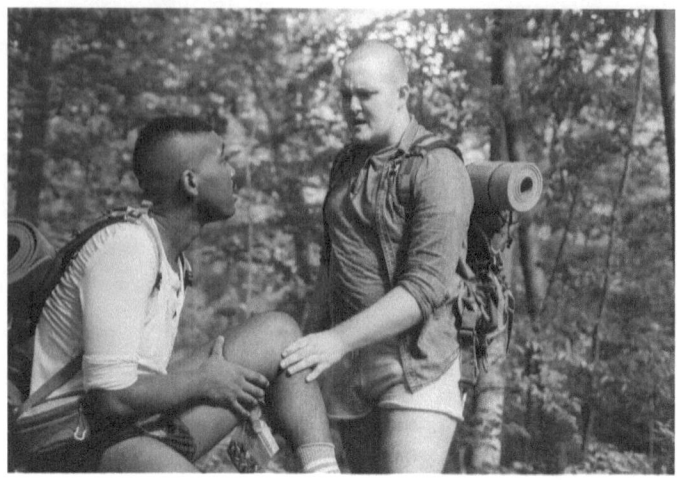

The comfort and ease of mind that a patient needs is something that as a healthcare person you must understand. The psychology of patients can range per patient and can be difficult to decode. With years of experience and most importantly with an urge to understand the situation, you will be able to help patients when they need your support the most.

HOW TO CALM YOUR PATIENT

Different patients will have different personalities, and it is up to you to figure out how to deal with each one of them. Sometimes the pain and the trauma caused by the illness or even accidents, for that matter, may cause disillusionment and can also give them a panic attack. In such a situation, you as their medical person can follow a few simple methods to help them calm down.

Be Engaging

As soon as the patient arrives or you meet the patient, engage them by asking them simple questions. Listen to them with attention and make them feel that they are heard. This can naturally calm down an anxious patient.

Give Relevant Information

While checking on the patient, you can talk and give relevant information about what the treatment will be like and how you plan to go ahead with it. Keeping them engaged in the process can help them think clearly. Ensure that the flow of communication between you and the patient is easy and without any confusion, as even a slight point of misunderstanding can cause panic and anxiety. Patience will be the key in dealing with patients who often experience some form of trauma or shock.

If you work for an organization, be aware of any

policies or clauses that may prevent you from indulging and disclosing specific information to your patients. You must always be careful of what extra, unnecessary information you might indulge in giving. While doing so, inquire about the patient's medical history. Do not coerce the patients; instead, give them ample time to answer your questions.

Do Not Complicate Things

Keep things simple by speaking to the patient rather than using medical jargon. By asking simple inquiries about how they feel and other health-related questions, you can divert your patient's thoughts from a state of anxiety, to one of stability. Your objective should be clear, and in any medical situation, it should be to make the patient feel better. Think with clarity while dealing with a case and take one step at a time. Examine every symptom and indicator before jumping to any conclusions. Utilize your expertise gained through experience, investigate all aspects of the situation, and then come to a decision to assist in the treatment of the issues.

Address Their Worries

Addressing their worries by asking them what they are fearing can help an anxious patient talk about their problems. By understanding their thoughts, you can give them sound advice and help them with their concerns. The most crucial skill is being a good listener. As a medical professional, you must always be aware of your patient's state of mind before beginning a treatment procedure. It is a natural process that when you address people's fears and conditions, you will be able to understand the situation and, as a result, it will be easier for you to solve the issue and keep the patient safe. More attention should be paid to what they are concerned about, and then a treatment plan should be devised accordingly.

Stay Calm

An anxious patient can have a panic attack if they realize that the medical practitioner is stressed. No matter how difficult you may find the situation and how complicated the case may look, ensure that in front of the patient, you do not lose your cool. Stay calm and make the patient realize that you are in a good mood. The confidence that you ooze out of your personality is what will help your patients feel safe and a sense of calm.

The self-assurance that you exude from your personality is what will make your patients feel secure and at ease. It's unusual for patients to function effectively in a confined, distracting environment. Having a calm approach to interacting with your patients can aid you in comprehending even the most difficult situations. Panic and hostility will not help you in a difficult situation. As a result, you must understand that by being calm, you will be able to treat your patients in a much better way.

Lighten Their Mood

If you find the patient is extremely tense, then you can ask them light questions that can help divert their mind to something else. Ask them about their hobbies and what they like to eat, etc. By creating such distractions, you can engage your patient even when they are in panic mode.

Empathize

Tell your patient that what they are feeling is

normal. Ask them to stay calm as that can help them get better soon.

Patients who feel that they are taken care of well seem to be much calmer during any medical procedures. Such an attitude can be a huge determining factor in how a person will recover during and after a treatment process.

Every case will be different in terms of the patient's behavior and receptive capability. You can use the following measures to find more information:

- Consider co-occurring disorders: While you attend to the patient analyze the situation and think if there could be anything they are not telling you. Ask questions gently and try to get as much information as you can.
- Immediately start considering any doubts that you feel regarding their present situation. If you have any concerns about the cause of the problem, make sure to note them down.
- Be mindful of situations that can take place later during or after the treatment

and make arrangements to have a smooth treatment process.

- Take their overall mental health into account: It is always wise to understand the mental health of a patient. Many times, patients tend to give a wrong narration of their injury or illness, and at times they can exaggerate situations. This can affect and have serious consequences on the treatment that you will provide. Be sure that what the patient is saying is correct, try to understand the state of mind of the patient by asking a few cross-questions, and then go ahead with the treatment accordingly.

- Medical history: Medical history is important and many people, unknowingly, fear talking about the medical issues they've had in the past. Figure out ways to ask them if they've had any particular medicine or previous symptoms. Be tricky but in a very subtle manner and get information on their health.

- Ask if they are taking any medication or under treatment for any other disease. This is because some medicines cannot be given at the same time and can cause serious reactions. Their present physical and mental health should be open to you before you start on your procedure to treat the patient. Every person responds to the same medication in different ways, be sure of what treatment you plan to give them and how they can deal with it.

ALLERGIES

Sometimes conditions that may look very serious may be a result of allergies that even the patients may not be aware of having. Understanding allergies in such a case can be very useful.

If you are in the wild, then your chances of encountering allergic reactions may be many.

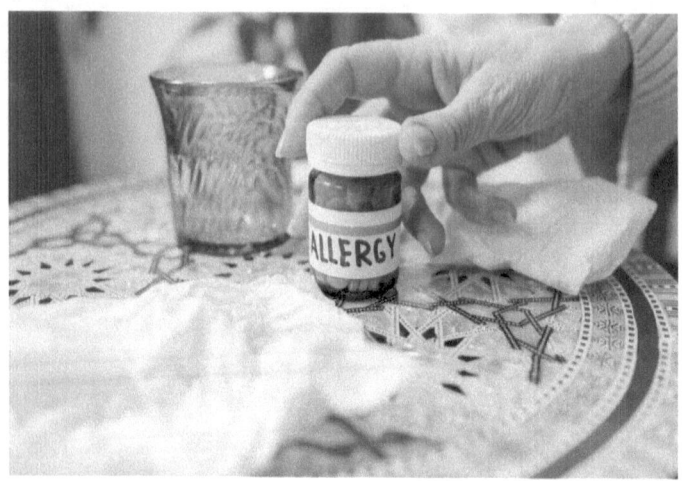

With the following information, you will be able to sail yourself through even in the toughest of allergic problems:

- Find out what you are allergic to. By identifying the root cause of your allergy, you can protect yourself and at the same time, can fight it more effectively. Some people are allergic to dust, pollen, grasses, weeds, certain plants, trees, oils, food, and even fruit.
- Develop a plan to protect yourself from allergies. If you get highly affected by pollen grains, then make sure you avoid outdoors during spring when there is a

huge rush of pollen grains being transported by bees and other insects. Keep your windows and doors at your home shut.

- Avoid eating food items that have an adverse reaction in your body.
- Clean yourself thoroughly to avoid any external dirt or allergic component attacking your system.
- Wear a mask if you have dust and pollen allergies.
- Inhalation treatment through steam can also be done to clean your nose pipes where allergens can be hidden.
- Try alternative methods to heal your allergy problems like acupuncture and other natural herbal remedies.

To counter allergies, you must be sure of your triggers. Once you're sure of what makes you sick, half your battle is already won. You can avoid whatever makes you allergic and stay safe in the long run.

DEALING WITH STINGS, BITES, AND ALL THINGS BUGS

The ecosystem is abundant with a wide range of insects and bugs. If you love the wild and are a regular wilderness explorer, then you must know by now that stings and bites can be some of the most common problems while out on an expedition.

In the US and surrounding regions, ticks, wasps, mosquitoes, bees, and even spiders and scorpions can be found in abundance. Every bite of these creatures is different and has a different result. Some just cause irritation whereas some are capable of spreading venom in the body.

It will be a wise decision to venture out in the wild with a few options in mind for dealing with such issues:

- Always carry a strong insect repellent.
- Choose a safe spot potentially free of harmful insects especially for a halt or a night stay.
- If a bee stings, then immediately remove the stinger. Use a tweezer for the process.
- Clean a bite or a sting area in the skin immediately with soap and water.

- Do not scratch the affected areas.
- Never go near a bee, hornet, or a wasp's nest. Keep in mind that some types of bees and wasps make nests in the ground.
- A cold compress or an ice pack will always help in such a situation. It can even help reduce swelling.
- For serious allergic reactions, make sure you carry your antiallergic medicine and shots.
- If the allergic reaction does not soothe even after an anti-allergic shot, then rush the patient to the nearest healthcare facility.

When you are on a hike in the outdoors, the chances are high that many insects like ticks and spiders can clutch in your clothes, and you may not even realize. Do not sleep with the clothes that you've traveled in through the woods. If changing is not possible, then dust your entire body with a piece of cloth.

Spider and scorpion stings can be fatal at times. When you encounter such a situation, first wash the affected area with antiseptic soap and water and then apply a cold compress. Observe if there are any symptoms like muscle spasm, nausea, vomiting, convulsions, and impaired speech and if so, do not wait any longer, rush the patient to the nearest medical center immediately.

SKIN ISSUES

Skin issues can be another problem while out in the woods. Refrain from touching plants that you've not been in contact with before. There are numerous plants out in the woods that can cause serious rashes and allergies to the skin.

Not just plants and insects, overexposure to the sun or the snow can cause the skin to burn. Always use a sunscreen lotion on your exposed skin even if there is no visible sun.

Carry anti-allergic medicines and skin-soothing creams that can cool your rashes and provide you relief from the constant itches and pain.

Cover your face with a light scarf while you are moving around the forest areas.

TRANSPORTING THE PATIENT

If you encounter any patient in the wild who has fallen from a cliff or just had a bad accident in the woods, do not move their body instantly. Injuries are not always visible and can be internal as well. It is your duty as a medical person to keep the patient as safe as possible in any given situation.

The first thought that will always come to your mind is to shift the patient to a stable and comfortable place for further treatment. Here are a few techniques that you can use to lift and safely move the patient:

- drags
- basic drag
- blanket drag
- backpack carry
- chair carry
- fireman's carry
- four-hand seat
- improvised harness carry
- papoose sling
- piggyback
- supported piggyback
- two-person carry
- wheelbarrow carry
- improvised litters

Apart from these techniques, you can use blankets and thick clothes to carry the patient by four people like a stretcher. Woods and long bamboo plants can be tied with each other to make stretchers. In the wild where there are no medical accessories available, if you have to rush the patient from a hill to the medical center, then you can use some of these methods to smoothly carry them without causing any further damage to their injury. Ensure that the patient is not jerked, pulled, or pushed during the process.

SERVING AS A NURSE

When you've made a decision and commitment to become a medical asset, you must always be mindful that emergencies can crop up at any time and can happen to anyone. Once you've taken up the role as a caregiver, it is your prerogative to be available for those in need around you.

There might be situations where you might be caught up with other priorities of your own, in such cases, make sure that you direct the patient to another trusted caregiver.

PROPER USE OF ANTIBIOTICS

Antibiotics have been mentioned a couple of times in this book and rightly so, as any survival kit will have its share of antibiotics. Antibiotics should be used as per a doctor's consultation and even if you decide to use them at your discretion, then listed below are a few dos and don'ts for the usage of antibiotics.

Dos

- Use antibiotics smartly and with caution.
- Consume them in correct doses and for the exact time period only. Do not stop taking them as soon as you feel better; finish the course as prescribed or directed.
- Consume only if needed.
- Antibiotics treat bacteria caused infections like whooping cough, strep throat, and urinary tract infections.

Don'ts

- Do not consume antibiotics regularly.
- Antibiotics do not work on cold

symptoms, sore throats, flu, and bronchitis.
- Antibiotics are not needed for sinus infections.

Make sure that you take antibiotics exactly as prescribed by your doctor. Do not self-medicate as that can cause more complications later on. Some side effects like rash, nausea, yeast infections, and diarrhea can be caused due to the usage of antibiotics. Make sure that you immediately call the doctor if the symptoms persist.

EMERGENCY CHILDBIRTH

Pregnancy and childbirth can be tricky situations if you are in the backcountry. Dealing with pregnancy is way easier than having to deal with delivering a sudden child out in the open. If you are trained and have knowledge about pregnancy-related concerns and childbirth, then you can very well save lives in an emergency. Here are some of the most important steps that you must take when you encounter a woman in labor:

- Immediately call 911 or any local emergency number.
- If you notice the pregnant woman's water is broken, and there is time for the medics to arrive, then lay her down in a comfortable place.
- Labor contractions can be long or short depending on the woman.
- If the woman says that she is getting cramps, then start preparing for the delivery process.
- Observe if the labor pressure is getting faster; faster means that the child is approaching.
- Maintain your cool and try to calm the woman by making her take long breaths.
- As the woman approaches the transitional phase, she will start making an effort to push naturally.
- Look into her vagina and check if the baby's head can be seen. Encourage her to take long breaths and to keep pushing.
- Ensure you support the head of the baby as it begins to come out. Once the head is out, the rest of the baby's body will easily follow.

- Be extra careful as the newborn will be slippery.
- As soon as the baby cries, keep the baby on the mother's chest and keep the child covered with something warm.
- The final and the most crucial step is to deal with the placenta. This is a vital part, as the placenta will take from 10 minutes to an hour to come out of the mother's body. With a little bit of pressure, the mother will push the placenta out.
- Firmly but with extra caution, massage her body slowly, making sure the bleeding stops.

Delivering a baby can be a difficult task, and it is advised not to practice this if you have no proper medical training. However, at times during emergencies, knowing about childbirth can help you in humongous ways.

Knowledge about various medical conditions can turn into a blessing if you can save someone's life. How you deal with an injured person or a person who is ill cannot just help you gain experience but can make you realize the importance of learning the knowledge of medicine.

Leave a 1-Click Review!

Customer reviews

⭐⭐⭐⭐⭐ 5 out of 5

3 global ratings

5 star	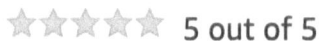	100%
4 star		0%
3 star		0%
2 star		0%
1 star		0%

⌄ How are ratings calculated?

Review this product

Share your thoughts with other customers

   Write a customer review

Other Titles!

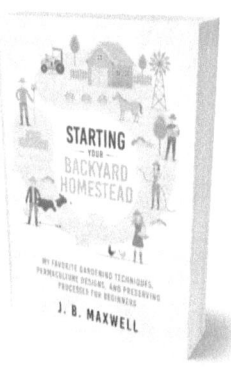

https://www.amazon.com/dp/B09PK252MF

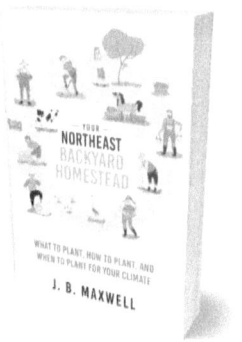

Northeast Backyard
Homestead

AFTERWORD

In a fast moving world like this, being a medical asset can make you highly relevant. It is a job that cannot just give you a good payoff but can be equally rewarding as well. The confidence that you can gain by becoming adept in knowing and understanding various concepts of medicine, from acupuncture and traditional medicines to herbal treatments, from survival strategies in the wild to basic medical knowledge including childbirth, can help you evolve in unimaginable ways.

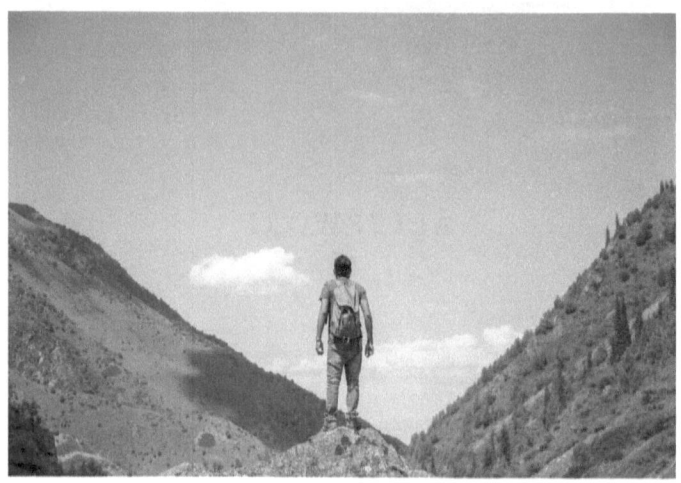

Your pursuit of medical education can help you have a successful prospect, making you useful in every place that you go. Whether you plan to work continuously as a medical practitioner or you want to venture out in the wild for a little longer, one thing that remains constant is the knowledge that can help you save your life as well as those around you.

Preparation is always good. You do not have to worry about preparing because something negative might happen. If that is your perspective, then that can attract a more negative vibe around you. Keep your focus on what you want and learn to face any difficulty. The goal is to become so competent, that even the most challenging times will crumble in the light of your knowledge.

There can be no virtue better than that of saving another's life. It is not just a job; the point remains that you are capable of saving people. Use your knowledge in the best possible way, and the contentment that you receive will be beyond any comparison.

Therefore, grab that first aid bag and begin your journey of becoming a medical asset. Think of all the lives that you will be able to save and the journeys that you can take in the wilderness without any fear. Your knowledge will become your confidence. No age is too young or too old to start a new journey or to gain a new education. Take a step forward, and the road ahead will all be yours!

REFERENCES

5 benefits of herbal medicine. (2020, May 22). Pinkham Medical. https://pinkhammedical.com/blog/5-benefits-of-herbal-medicine/

5 reasons why we need healthcare professionals now more than ever. (2020, November 4). The George Washington University School of Business. https://healthcaremba.gwu.edu/blog/5-reasons-why-we-need-healthcare-professionals-now-more-than-ever/

10 health issues caused by bad oral health. (2021, October 11). Absolute Dental. https://www.absolut-edental.com/blog/10-health-issues-caused-by-bad-oral-health/

12 natural ways to defeat allergies. (2021, February

18). WebMD. https://www.webmd.com/allergies/allergy-education-17/slideshow-natural-relief

50 mind-blowing true survival stories (hiking, kidnapping, lost at sea, plane crashes and more). (2020, June 30). Trek Baron. https://trekbaron.com/survival-stories/

A brief history of medicine. (2013, August 8). FutureLearn. https://www.futurelearn.com/info/courses/study-medicine/0/steps/147884

Altitude sickness. (2020, September 23). Cleveland Clinic. https://my.clevelandclinic.org/health/diseases/15111-altitude-sickness

Andrea, S. (2017). *Snow covered mountain during sunrise.* Pexels. [Image]. https://www.pexels.com/photo/snow-covered-mountain-during-sunrise-618833/

Barbosa, C. (2019). *Close-up photo of woman with her eyes closed holding her forehead.* Pexels. [Image]. https://www.pexels.com/photo/close-up-photo-of-woman-with-her-eyes-closed-holding-her-forehead-2023128/

Basic first aid skills—identifying and addressing altitude sickness. (2016, October 10). Adventure equipped. https://www.adventuremedicalkits.-

com/blog/2016/10/basic-first-aid-skills-identify-ing-and-addressing-altitude-sickness/

Bedosky, L. (2021, November 5). *8 ways to keep your immune system healthy*. EverydayHealth. https://www.everydayhealth.com/columns/white-seeber-grogan-the-remedy-chicks/ten-simple-natural-ways-to-boost-immune-system/

Biological hazard. (2021). In *Wikipedia*. https://en.wikipedia.org/wiki/Biological_hazard

Bones, muscles, and joints. (2012, October). Rady Children's Hospital, San Diego. https://www.rchs-d.org/health-articles/bones-muscles-and-joints-2/

Bones, muscles and joints. (2021, September). Healthdirect. https://www.healthdirect.gov.au/bones-muscles-and-joints

Brazier, Y. (2020, November 29). *Anatomy: A brief introduction*. MedicalNewsToday. https://www.med-icalnewstoday.com/articles/248743

Breathing difficulties—first aid. (2021, November 20). MedlinePlus. https://medlineplus.gov/ency/ar-ticle/000007.htm

Buer, S. (2016, June 3). *27 considerations for a wilderness first aid kit*. NOLS Blog. https://blog.nols.e-du/2016/06/03/27-considerations-for-a-first-aid-kit

Burns, L. (2009, November 5). *First aid in the era*

of biohazards. Industrial Safety & Hygiene News. https://www.ishn.com/articles/88912-first-aid-in-the-era-of-biohazards#:~:text=Use%20germicidal%20towelettes%20or%20bleach

Chemical emergency preparedness. (2018). American Red Cross. https://www.redcross.org/get-help/how-to-prepare-for-emergencies/types-of-emergencies/chemical-emergency.html

Chemical hazard. (2021). In *Wikipedia.* https://en.wikipedia.org/wiki/Chemical_hazard

Chronic fatigue syndrome. (2020, September 24). Mayo Clinic. https://www.mayoclinic.org/diseases-conditions/chronic-fatigue-syndrome/symptoms-causes/syc-20360490

Cormier, S. (2017, April 18). *Disaster preparedness: 5 key components to effective emergency management.* HealthcareDive. https://www.healthcaredive.com/news/disaster-preparedness-5-key-compo-nents-to-effective-emergency-management/440672/

cottonbro. (2017). *Man putting on coveralls.* Pexels. [Image]. https://www.pexels.com/photo/man-putting-on-coveralls-3951417/

cottonbro. (2020). *Woman in white shirt holding silver pin.* Pexels. [Image]. https://www.pexels.com/photo/fashion-man-people-woman-5721551/

cottonbro. (2021). *Person holding allergy medicine bottle.* Pexels. [Image]. https://www.pexels.com/photo/person-holding-allergy-medicine-bottle-6865181/

Decker, S. (2018, June 5). *Into the woods: Top tips for wilderness medicine.* AAFP. https://www.aafp.org/news/blogs/freshperspectives/entry/20180605fp-wilderness.html

Frostbite. (2021, October 9). Mayo Clinic. https://www.mayoclinic.org/diseases-conditions/frostbite/symptoms-causes/syc-20372656

Gómez, O. (2018). *Man on top of mountain.* Pexels. [Image]. https://www.pexels.com/photo/man-on-top-of-mountain-840667/

Grabowska, K. (2020). *Crop unrecognizable male doctor with stethoscope.* Pexels. [Image]. https://www.pexels.com/photo/crop-unrecognizable-male-doctor-with-stethoscope-4021775/

Grabowska, K. (2021, January 28) *photo-of-a-dentist-demonstrating-how-to-brush-teeth.* Pexels. [Image]. https://www.pexels.com/photo/photo-of-a-dentist-demonstrating-how-to-brush-teeth-6627313/

Herbs to support healthy female hormone balance through all life stage. (2021, September 17). Gaia Herbs. https://www.gaiaherbs.com/blogs/seeds-of-knowledge/herbs-to-support-female-hormone-balance-through-all-life-stages

Home remedies for a sprained ankle. (2019, May 17). Top 10 Home Remedies. https://www.top10homeremedies.com/home-remedies/home-remedies-sprained-ankle.html

Home remedies: What works? (2021, February 18). WebMD. https://www.webmd.com/balance/ss/slideshow-home-remedies

How does naturopathic medicine lower health care costs? (n.d.). Institute for Natural Medicine. https://naturemed.org/faq/faq-how-does-naturopathic-medicine-lower-health-care-costs/

Hyponatremia. (2020, May 23). MayoClinic. https://www.mayoclinic.org/diseases-conditions/hyponatremia/symptoms-causes/syc-20373711

Hypothermia. (2020, April 18). Mayo Clinic. https://www.mayoclinic.org/diseases-conditions/hypothermia/diagnosis-treatment/drc-20352688

Immovable joint. (2021, June 28). Biology Online. https://www.biologyonline.com/dictionary/immovable-joint

Insomnia. (2016, October 15). Mayo Clinic.

https://www.mayoclinic.org/diseases-conditions/insomnia/symptoms-causes/syc-20355167

Jaspers, E. (2020, April 5). *Adaptability: When change is the only constant.* WeAreBrain. https://wearebrain.com/blog/our-company/adaptability-when-change-is-the-only-constant/

Khongchum, C. (2020). *Photo of female scientist working on laboratory*. Pexels. [Image]. https://www.pexels.com/photo/photo-of-female-scientist-working-on-laboratory-3938023/

Kim, J.H. (2018, July 2). Three principles for radiation safety: Time, distance, and shielding. *The Korean Journal of Pain*, 31(3), 145-146. https://www.ncbi.nlm.nih.gov/pmc/articles/PMC6037814/

Kisan, R., Sujan, M., Adoor, M., Raghavendra, R., Nalini, A., Kutty, B., Chindanda Murthy, B., Raju, TR., & Sathyaprabha, T. (2014). Effect of Yoga on migraine: A comprehensive study using clinical profile and cardiac autonomic functions. *International Journal of Yoga*, 7(2), 126-132. https://doi.org/10.4103/0973-6131.133891

Kuballa, J. (2018, February 4). *18 remedies to get rid of headaches naturally.* Healthline. https://www.healthline.com/nutrition/headache-remedies

Lipman, G. S., Eifling, K. P., Ellis, M. A., Gaudio,

F. G., Otten, E. M., & Grissom, C. K. (2014). Wilderness Medical Society practice guidelines for the prevention and treatment of heat-related illness: 2014 Update. *Wilderness & Environmental Medicine*, 25(4), 355–365. https://doi.org/10.1016/j.wem.2014.07.017

Macwelch, T. (2021, April 20). *Survival skills: How to make a mud cast in 4 steps*. OutdoorLife. https://www.outdoorlife.com/blogs/survivalist/survival-skills-how-make-mud-cast-4-steps/

Myers, T., & Hoffman, M. (2015, April 29). Hiker fatality from severe hyponatremia in Grand Canyon National Park. *Wilderness and Environmental Medicine*, 26(3), 371-374. https://www.wemjournal.org/article/S1080-6032(15)00117-9/fulltext

Monstera. (2021). *World map made of tablets and capsules and little lock*. Pexels. [Image]. https://www.pexels.com/photo/world-map-made-of-tablets-and-capsules-and-little-lock-7411935/

Naturopathy. (2021). In *Wikipedia*. https://en.wikipedia.org/wiki/Naturopathy

Naturopathy less expensive than conventional medicine in the long run. (2020, January 9). Express Healthcare. https://www.expresshealthcare.in/interviews/naturopathy-less-expensive-than-conventional-medicine-in-the-long-run/416093/

nhinkle. (2015, December 6). *How to create a cast or splint to aid a broken bone?* [Online forum post]. StackExchange. https://outdoors.stackexchange.com/questions/10145/how-to-create-a-cast-or-splint-to-aid-a-broken-bone

Nierenberg, C. (2016, October 27). *7 strategies for outdoor lovers with seasonal allergies.* Livescience. https://www.livescience.com/56607-outdoor-lovers-seasonal-allergies-tips.html

Ogino, K. (2020). *Tourists talking to each other in forest.* Pexels. [Image]. https://www.pexels.com/photo/tourists-talking-to-each-other-in-forest-5064636/

Ong, C. (2015, January 9). *5 benefits of strategic planning.* Envisio. https://envisio.com/blog/benefits-of-strategic-planning/

Pixabay. (2016, December 21). *Emergency signage.* Pexels. [Image]. https://www.pexels.com/photo/ambulance-architecture-building-business-263402/

Ponsford, S. (2017, December 14). *How to treat a toothache at home.* Medical News Today. https://www.medicalnewstoday.com/articles/320315

Productions, R. (2021a). *Paramedic performing CPR.* Pexels. [Image]. https://www.pexels.com/photo/paramedic-performing-cpr-6520071/

Productions, R. (2021b). *Person applying bandage*

on another person's hand. Pexels. [Image]. https://www.pexels.com/photo/person-applying-bandage-on-another-person-s-hand-6519905/

Protecting yourself from radiation. (2021, May 21). EPA. https://www.epa.gov/radiation/protecting-yourself-radiation

RF._.studio (2019, October 10)). Photo of woman studying anatomy. Pexels. [Image]. https://www.pexels.com/photo/photo-of-woman-studying-anatomy-3059750/

RF._.studio (2020, February 28). Unrecognizable African American scientist studying anatomy with tablet. Pexels. [Image]. https://www.pexels.com/photo/unrecognizable-african-american-scientist-studying-anatomy-with-tablet-3825539/

Ryser, S. (2019, March 7). Basic first aid skills everyone should learn. Idaho Medical Academy. https://www.idahomedicalacademy.com/basic-first-aid-skills-everyone-should-learn/

Sarnacki, A. (2019, September 5). 10 medicinal plants for your natural first aid kit. Hello Homestead. https://hellohomestead.com/10-medicinal-plants-for-your-natural-first-aid-kit/

Schimelpfenig, T. (2020, September 18). How to treat insect bites and stings. REI CO OP.

https://www.rei.com/learn/expert-advice/how-to-treat-insect-bites-and-stings.html

Shah, N., Hussain, S., Cooke, M., O'Hara, J. P., & Mellor, A. (2015). Wilderness medicine at high altitude: Recent developments in the field. *Open Access Journal of Sports Medicine*, 6, 319–328. https://doi.org/10.2147/OAJSM.S89856

ShemSeger. (2015, December 4). *How to create a cast or splint to aid a broken bone?* [Online forum post]. StackExchange. https://outdoors.stackexchange.com/questions/10145/how-to-create-a-cast-or-splint-to-aid-a-broken-bone

Shuraev, Y. (2021). *Person walking on snow covered field while wearing cold wear*. Pexels. [Image]. https://www.pexels.com/photo/person-walking-on-snow-covered-field-while-wearing-cold-wear-7042404/

Sieroslawska, A. (2021, October 28). *Bones*. Kenhub. https://www.kenhub.com/en/library/anatomy/bones

Stickler, T. (2020, June 4). *Migraine herbal home remedies from around the world*. Healthline. https://www.healthline.com/health/migraine-herbal-home-remedies-from-around-the-world

Tankilevitch, P. (2020). *Person holding thermometer*. Pexels. [Image]. https://www.pexels.-

com/photo/person-holding-thermometer-3873188/

The Editors of Encyclopedia Britannica. (2020, September 8). *Pulmonary circulation*. Britannica. https://www.britannica.com/science/pulmonary-circulation

The five worst nuclear disasters in history. (2014, July 30). Process Industry Forum. https://www.processindustryforum.com/energy/five-worst-nuclear-disasters-history

The human body. (2020, December 2). Healthline. https://www.healthline.com/human-body-maps#reproductive-system-female

Thomas, A. (2012, April 18). *Medicine and surgery before 1800—the Enlightenment*. homeobook. https://www.homeobook.com/medicine-and-surgery-before-1800-the-enlightenment/

Thompson, W., Underwood, E.A., Richardson, R., Guthrie, D., Rhodes, P., & The Editors of Encyclopedia Britannica. (2020, August 27). *History of Medicine*. Britannica. https://www.britannica.com/science/history-of-medicine/Traditional-medicine-and-surgery-in-Asia

Tips to get rid of a headache. (2015, December 29). WebMD. https://www.webmd.com/migraines-headaches/5-ways-to-get-rid-of-headache

Tomczak, M. (2004). *Lecture 9: The quest for health, the dawn of medical science.* Incois.gov.in. https://incois.gov.in/Tutor/science+society/lectures/lecture9.html

Torn ligament—causes, symptoms, and treatment. (2010, March 17). HealthHearty. https://healthhearty.com/torn-ligament

Types of bone. (n.d.). Lumen. https://courses.lumenlearning.com/wm-biology2/chapter/types-of-bone/

Types of fractures. (2019, March 28). Complete Care. https://www.visitcompletecare.com/blog/types-of-fractures/

Urinary tract infections. (2010). https://www.kidney.org/sites/default/files/uti.pdf

user5330. (2015, December 6). *How to create a cast or splint to aid a broken bone?* [Online forum post]. StackExchange. https://outdoors.stackexchange.com/questions/10145/how-to-create-a-cast-or-splint-to-aid-a-broken-bone

Vaitkevich, N. (2021). *Flat lay photo of alternative medicines.* Pexels. [Image]. https://www.pexels.com/photo/flat-lay-photo-of-alternative-medicines-7615463/

Van Sloun, N. (2015, November 28). *Natural remedies for everyday illness.* AllinaHealth. https://

www.allinahealth.org/healthysetgo/heal/natural-remedies-for-everyday-illnesses

Wachtel-Galor, S. & Benzie, F. (2011). *Chapter 1: Herbal medicine.* NCBI. https://www.ncbi.nlm.nih.gov/books/NBK92773/

Welby, M. (2020, March 17). *The anxious patient: How to calm a patient down to improve care.* Wolters Kluwer. https://www.wolterskluwer.com/en/expert-insights/the-anxious-patient-how-to-calm-a-patient-down-to-improve-care

Welz, A. N., Emberger-Klein, A., & Menrad, K. (2018). Why people use herbal medicine: Insights from a focus-group study in Germany. *BMC Complementary and Alternative Medicine,* 18(92). https://doi.org/10.1186/s12906-018-2160-6

What is a biohazard? Six examples. (2021, April 9). Helix Solutions. https://www.helixsolutions.net.au/news-and-resources/article/what-is-a-biohazard-six-examples

What is natural medicine? (2021, April 26). Health Times. https://healthtimes.com.au/hub/natural-medicine/72/guidance/ht1/what-is-natural-medicine/2115/

What to do in an emergency. (2020, February 13). NHSinform. https://www.nhsinform.scot/illnesses-

and-conditions/heart-and-blood-vessels/heart-emergencies/what-to-do-in-an-emergency

Who should choose a Healthcare MBA? (2017, October 26). The George Washington University School of Business. https://healthcaremba.gwu.edu/

World Health Organization. (2019). *WHO global report on traditional and complementary medicine 2019.* https://www.who.int/traditional-complementary-integrative-medicine/WhoGlobalReportOnTraditionalAndComplementaryMedicine2019.pdf

Worldspectrum. (2018, May 23). *Beige python on brown branch of tree.* Pexels. [Image]. https://www.pexels.com/photo/beige-python-on-brown-branch-of-tree-110819/

Yeast infection in men (balanitis). (2017, June 7). STD. https://www.std-gov.org/stds/yeast_in_man.htm